SOME ACCOUNT OF THE GENERAL AND MEDICAL TOPOGRAPHY OF AJMEER

SOME ACCOUNT OF THE GENERAL AND MEDICAL TOPOGRAPHY OF AJMEER

ROBERT HAMILTON IRVINE

GYAN

Published by

GYAN

Gyan Publishing House
5, Ansari Road
Daryaganj, New Delhi-110002
Phone: 011-47034999, 9811692060
E-mail: books@gyanbooks.com

Distribution Network
gyanbooks.com
India, USA, Canada, UK, Australia

ISBN: 978-93-6433-668-0 (PB)
First Published, 1841

2nd Impression 2024

Printed at: Gyan Press, Delhi.

SOME ACCOUNT OF THE GENERAL AND MEDICAL TOPOGRAPHY OF AJMEER

AUTHOR: ROBERT HAMILTON IRVINE

SOME ACCOUNT

OF THE

GENERAL AND MEDICAL TOPOGRAPHY

OF

AJMEER.

BY

ASSISTANT-SURGEON ROBERT HAMILTON IRVINE, M.D.

PRINTED BY ORDER OF THE GOVERNMENT.

CALCUTTA:
W. THACKER AND CO., ST. ANDREW'S LIBRARY.
1841.

SOME ACCOUNT

OF THE

GENERAL AND MEDICAL TOPOGRAPHY

OF

AJMEER.

In drawing up the subsequent remarks on the Topography of Ajmeer, I am more actuated by the desire of strictly conforming to the wishes of the Government, than by the conviction of having any facts of peculiar interest to communicate. The thought indeed of the, perhaps apparent, barrenness of subject, in relation to the nature of the country to be discussed, might otherwise have deterred me from commencing the task imposed. I hope, therefore, that I may obtain every indulgence for defects, if not positive approbation for merits. General Description.

The term Ajmeer, taken in the broadest acceptation, applies to the whole of Rajpootanah, being the more ancient appellation; taken however in the modern proper sense, Ajmeer designates only the city so called and the district attached. Ancient Province of Ajmeer.

The province of Ajamida, Ajmeer, Rajpootanah, or Rajasthan, was anciently situated principally between the 22nd and 30th degrees of north latitude, and from the 69th to the 78th degree of east longitude, and embraced a superficial area of 350,000 square miles. But, this space, during the superposition of minor Mahommedan dynasties, was considerably circumscribed. Rajasthan (or the abode of Rajpoots) is the now correct denomination of this part of India: and in the familiar dialect of these countries, is termed Rajwarra or Raethana: and by the British, Rajpootanah, to denote the Rajpoot principalities.

According to this division, the Sinde river in Malwa marked the eastern boundary, as did the Indus (or great Sinde) that to the west. The included space was Rajpootanah, in the acmè of Rajpoot splendour, formed by the kingdoms of the various Rajpoot princes, who, at the heads of their respective tribes, had conquered the aborigines, and seized on the land with the hand of power. Subsequently, this space was much diminished by the inroads of the Mahommedan conquerors; both by the fate of battles, and extensive concessions of land, made by the Rajpoots, to avoid collision with the Islamites. In this way the monarchies of Maudoo and Ahmedabad arose on the ruins of Dhar and Auhulwarra Patun, which were wrested from their Rajpoot possessors.

It would appear, that east of the Sinde in Malwa no really Rajpoot state was ever established; for even those Hindoos to the eastward of this river, calling themselves Chuttrees, and claiming privileges as such, are not considered of pure blood by either the rulers or commonalty of Rajwarra, from association with whom they are excluded in all points relating to caste.

Modern Ajmeer. The present province of Rajpootanah is very irregular in form, and the extreme points appear to be 29° 30″ 0′ and 23° 15″ 0′ north latitude, and from 70° 30″ 0′ to 77° 15″ 0′ east longitude.

Different States The different states comprised, are Mewar or Oodipoor, Marwar or Jodpoor, Jaepoor or Ambĕr, Beekaneer, Jessulmeer, Kotah, Boondi, Kishengurh, Sirohie, and (in medio almost) Ajmeer and Mairwarra districts under British rule.

General Appearance. From the very great extent of Rajpootanah, a very great variety of features, diversifies the surface of the country. The most elevated point is Mount Aboo, an insulated mountain in Mewar, and the highest in Hindusthan proper, being nearly 5,000 feet above the level of the sea: and towering about 1,500 feet above the Aravulli range of hills. Next, in point of elevation are the Aravulli, the highest of the peaks being 3,500 feet above the level of the sea. No other ranges of hills present any great elevations. The highest of the remaining elevations are in the vicinity of Ajmeer and Mairwarra. Taraghur, near the former city, being about 1,000 feet above the plains around, and 2,000 feet above the sea. The highest of the peaks of the Mairwarra ranges being somewhat less. The plateau of central India, called by the natives Patàr (equivalent in meaning to table-land), is embraced within these regions, and extends from Jawud to Shahabad in Harowtee, forming a level (interspersed with hills) and is very generally from 1,500 to 1,800 feet above the level of the sea. This table-land prevents the chief streams of Mewar (or Med-pet) from directly joining the Chumbul river; those which flow from the Aravulli range, running towards the Beris and Bunas, with which they chiefly unite. The central plateau itself abounds in minor ranges of hills: and is also in some places divided by narrow steep-sided valleys. It appears from the best surveys, that the lowest points in these regions, are at least 1,000 feet above the sea level. In traversing Harowtee, on the eastern frontier there is an abrupt descent from the plateau to the level of the river Sinde: from Kotah to Rampoora and Ruttunghur a considerable ascent takes place: thus forming three "steppes" in succession.

A line drawn from Oodipoor to Kotra on the Betwa is nearly six geographical degrees in extent, and at a short distance from and parallel to the tropical line, passes over a country of the greatest interest, being highly diversified, both in inhabitants, and productions of soil, either vegetable or hidden in the ground. This line nearly would bisect the central land (or media-desa) of Rajasthan.

The eastern portion of Rajpootanah is defined by the course of the Chumbul and its tributary streams till confluence with the Jumna. The western portion being those regions west of the Aravulli range. The southern division extends to Malwa, in some places bounded by the Vindhya chain, or by the spurs thrown out from those hills. The northern division is bounded by Hurreeanah, Mooltan and the Delhi territory.

Diversity of Climate. In this immense tract of country, a very great diversity of climate is observed.

Partial Civilization. The greater portion is very little civilized: and some parts have no claim to be even so designated.

From Aboo a space of nearly sixty miles passing through Ogema, Punurwa and Meerpoor westward towards Sirohie is a continued series of steep hills and jungles of an almost impenetrable nature, as far as the junction with the plains of Marwar. This space is inhabited by communities of the aboriginal races (chiefly Bheels) living in a savage and independent state, owning no paramount power, but having hereditary leaders styled "Rawuts." Of the natural history of this tract nothing is known, no European having penetrated far enough for observation. Even our troops, occasionally sent on service, have generally been prevented by the nature of the country from effecting the object in view.

From Komulmēr, in Mewar, the Aravulli range runs north towards Ajmeer, near which its tabular form is lost, and it breaks into lofty ridges running through Shekawattie, Ulwer, and terminating in the low Mewattie hills near Delhi.

Mairwarra. The whole space, from Komulmēr to Ajmeer in this range, is termed Mairwarra, inhabited by a race of hill men, of peculiar habits, termed "Mairs" (from mēr, signifying "hill"): this space is about 60 miles in length, and averages from six miles (the narrowest) to 15 miles (the greatest) breadth: containing a great number of villages. The people are warlike, and were habitual plunderers.

Beawr. Part of this tract is now a British district, under the admirable rule of Captain Dixon, the Superintendent of Beawr; where a fine corps absorbs the plundering energies of the Mairs, and improvements and cultivation now proceed in all directions.

Northern Division. The northern division of this province, comprehending Beekaneer, and the neighbouring districts, is a barren unfertile plain, bare of trees, and almost destitute of rivers and rivulets, and but very thinly inhabited.

The more central portion, which includes Jodpoor and Jaepoor, is more hilly, and is better supplied with water, yet seldom in sufficient quantity for wet crops. The soil is often of a remarkably saline nature, and there are numerous salt springs, and some large salt lakes : both salt and saltpetre are spontaneously produced.

The southern division is of an excellent soil; some parts are very fertile; and abound in hills and extensive plains, beautifully wooded and watered by numerous streams. Southern Division.

Of the rivers, the Chumbul and Bunas are the chief; the smaller rivers Beris, Bunas, Khataserie, Khari and the Dye, all unite with the great Bunas to the eastward; to the westward, the numerous small streams, that water the rich district of Godwar, unite with the salt river, or Looni, and mark the line of the desert; of these streams the chief are the Sookri and the Bandi; most of the remainder not being perennial, but depending on atmospheric causes for a supply, and are commonly known under the general appellation of "raye," or "torrents;" most of these, by depositing during floods, a quantity of alluvial earth, enrich portions of the otherwise barren silicious soil. Rivers.

The Aravulli and subordinate ranges, probably abound in metallic ores: and in many places mines are now worked but not to the extent of former periods. Tin and silver were once found and worked; and, now, copper, lead and iron are abundantly produced. Metallic Ores.

Of these regions the Patàr is very remarkable, consisting generally of vast plains of horizontal stratification, with numerous ridges of hills rising to considerable elevations, and also valleys of considerable depth, with very perpendicular walls, cut through the superior stratas: the surface and hills, even where most stony, are beautifully wooded. Table-land.

This plateau appears to be erroneously described by Todd as of trap formation: which error probably arose, from the stratified sandstone, of which the plateau is formed, jutting out in a graduated or terrace-like way, in places where the strata have been ruptured, or cut through, to form valleys, or the courses of rivers: this is the only way in which the term "trap" can be applied to these strata, from the meaning of the word "trappa" (in Sweedish "a stair"). Trap, in the proper geological acceptation, being a natural family of rocks, having a tendency to assume a columnar formation, or to divide into steps forming natural terraces, *abounding in horneblende and augite*, and being generally of a greenish or blackish colour, and occurring in the primary, transition and tertiary formations: it is therefore quite evident that the term does not apply to the plateau of central India; which consists, excepting in the ridges of hills, of horizontal strata of silicious sandstone of the variegated variety, in thick strata split in various directions by deep fissures, generally at right angles and continuous to great depths, as becomes especially evident on inspecting the banks of the rivers. The sandstone is generally massive; but, is often split into slabs, and in some places becomes sandstone slate: it varies in colour from pure white to pinkish or brown, and is often streaked: and contains nodules and irregular fragments of iron ore, quartz, and jasper, in many places. The third variety of sandstone, or pure free-stone, is not found in the many parts of the Patàr that I have examined. It seems therefore evident that the Patàr is of the variegated sandstone (or tertiary) formation.

The geological and mineralogical remarks made by Colonel Todd, are often inaccurate. Thus the bed of the Chumbul is described as shewing "*milk-white trap*:" whereas the substance meant is quartz rock, which occurs abundantly in the bed of the Chumbul, below the sandstone strata, and varies from white to grey, massive and semi-transparent: similar quartzoze sandstone also abounds, one kind of which is very fine-grained, compact, hard, white, and opaque, of which the images at Barolli in Mewar are formed.

Todd also describes the Jain temple at Ajmeer as being constructed of "limestone:" whereas, the material is a fine-grained pure silicious sandstone, coloured yellow by iron : in the same way, black amorphous schorl is described as "bicullite."

The surface of the plateau is very unequally divided, and is continually alternating in character between a tabular form and clustering ridges : the plains, however, as before stated, being often very extensive ; the general elevation is higher than the summits of the Vindhya ranges, and on a level with the valley of Oodipoor and the base of the Aravulli.

There appear two distinctly marked declivities or slopes in central India : one from the Aravulli to the Betwa in Bundlekhund from west to east : and the other extending from the Vindhya mountains to the Jumna, from south to north. Natural Division.

To the westward of the Aravulli, extend the Rajpoot principalities of Jodpoor, Jessulmeer and Beekaneer, each forming part of the Thul or desert, which stretches from the Aravulli to the banks of the Indus. The Looni, or salt river, enriches the best portion of the Jodpoor territory, and marks the line of ever shifting sand (called "Maroo'-sthuli," or region of death) forming the plain of Marwar. The greater portion of these countries are arid in the highest degree, nearly destitute of trees, and the little water possessed is often of a saline nature ; they are in fact chiefly sandy plains ; but, the worst portion of the sandy desert commences beyond the frontiers of these principalities, to the north-westward. Nearly all this portion of territory is incumbent upon a sandstone foundation ; the deep wells generally penetrating to it. Desert.

From this description it is evident, that Rajpootanah, from the great extent, but chiefly from physical causes, possesses a very great variety of climates, by which the health of the inhabitants is much influenced. The diseases of an epidemic nature, by which they are attacked, vary extremely in frequency of occurrence and severity of type. Variety of Climate.

The level of this province varies from 1,000 to 2,000 feet above the level of the sea: the average temperature is Level.

therefore much modified, and generally greatly lower, than the latitude would indicate. The surface of the land, and the quantity of water present are extremely various: ranging from the most extensive sandy plains, almost destitute of water, to the deepest black loamy soils well watered, and retentive of moisture, and abounding in the most luxuriant vegetation.

As a general rule, the most desert portions are the healthiest, and liable to the mildest periodical diseases: whilst the most luxuriantly cultivated and the jungly portions are in every respect the reverse.

After this broad outline of the superficial aspect of Rajpootanah, I shall proceed shortly to describe the more particular attribute of each individual state, and shall conclude with the district of Ajmeer.

BEEKANEER.

Ancient Extent. This principality is described in the Aiyeen Akbary, as a Sircar of Marwar in the Soobah of Ajmeer; but very little seems to have been known about it at that time, except that it had been under the dominion of Khutres for some ages. This want of information, on the part of Abul Fuzul, probably arose from the merely nominal way in which the greater part of these states were subjected to the Mussulman yoke.

Modern. Beekaneer extends from 27½° to 29½° north latitude, and from 72½° to 79½° east longitude: the extreme length is from Beethnôk or Guriala, near Girrajsir, north-eastward, to near Bhutnēr, being 150 miles: and the extreme breadth from Poogul, south-eastward to near Ladnoo, or from Unoopghur south-eastward to near Chooroo, 100 miles; giving an area of about 13,500 square miles.

Aborigines. The aborigines are called Bhoomias (from "Bhoom," "the soil") and are the Getae, Jits, or Jauts, in greatest numbers: the Dhers, next: and after them the Aheiries. The Dhers and Aheiries (*very different from the aheer* or *gaowala* tribe) are both "mileetch," or lowest castes. The Dhers worship Ramdeojee (a "towar" Rajpoot saint;) they eat almost all animals that die naturally; but it is a curious fact, that they will neither keep nor eat tame or wild hogs: holding the latter even abominable, while their high caste Rajpoot masters consider the wild hog a great delicacy. The Aheiries are only a little less impure than the Dhers: they worship Paboojee (a Rhatore Rajpoot saint).

Ruler, Raja Ruttun Singh, Rhatore. Ruler

Tribes now inhabiting. Rajpoots; chiefly of the Rhatore tribe, then of the Sankla and Solankhie tribes, and a few of the immigrated Cuchwaha tribe, all of the Suriyavansa, or race of the sun. There are also a good many of the Bhattie tribe of Rajpoots, of the Indu or Soomvansa, or race of the moon. Tribes.

The brahmuns, are of the Pokhurna, Gour, Diva, Parik, Sikawar and Goozurgour tribes.

There are also "dacôt brahmuns," a begging tribe, who are descended from the union of a brahmun with one of the *Aheer* or cowkeeping caste: they eat impurely, and are despised by regular brahmuns: they will not work: they beg chiefly on Saturday: pretend to astrology: and receive impure articles (as oil, &c.) in charity.

There are also a few "boora brahmuns," who are a similarly degraded caste: they are much feared: they attend near the houses of the dying, especially of rich people; but are never admitted within the apartments, being dreaded, shunned and detested: they assert a claim to the clothes, lotah and bedding of the dead. The superstitious natives imagine that the "boora brahmun" possesses some power of causing misfortunes. This tribe daily prays for a "*fat subject*," with certain ceremonies, in the following words;

Aj, Mata, marro mota,
Tub moojh ko mila rota!

Oh! Mata, fat and rich ones slay,
To grant me food and clothes this day.

This people is rather numerous in Rajpootanah, and forms the terror of fat seths and bunyas, especially if one be met with in the morning.

The bunyas are of the Uggurwallah, Oswar, Suraogee, Maiserie, and Khutree, all, rich or poor, of the many ramifications of the "byess."

The cultivators are chiefly Jauts, then Chumars and Raegurs; a few Goozurs, are chiefly shepherds; and a good many Aheiries and Dhers. The whole tribes also, whether brahmuns or Rajpoots or otherwise, often become husbandmen by necessity, and many are always so.

A few Aheers or gaowalas, (cowkeepers) attend as personal servants on the princes. This tribe is most numerous in the Dukhan.

Weavers. These are chiefly Dhers; but there are also a few Joolahuhs, Mussulmanis.

Lohars. A peculiar small tribe exists, in this principality, which is migratory from village to village. They are said to have been formerly Rajpoots, who on the conquest of Cheetore by the Mahommedans, formed part of the garrison, and being violently assailed, and threatened with death, threw down their arms, declaring that they were Lohars; hence they became outcasts from their more brave companions, and have ever since been workers in iron. They travel about in small carts from village to village with their families, and are often seen in Rajwarra.

A few carpenters are scattered over the country; and the same is the case with the oilmen, goldsmiths, and the braziers.

A good many barbers are found: as they not only dress the hair of the Rajpoots, but can prepare food for the Rajpoot, who can eat from their hands, and on this account they are often kept: and they may cook even for the Rajpoot princes, as well as take care of the person.

Bards are numerous: and act as recorders of events: and, from their sacred character, as protectors and guides to caravans, or travellers.

Hindoo camel breeders, are very numerous: they attend the herds of camels: and also accompany them when employed on the road.

Of tailors there are a few of Hindoo faith.

Cow and sheep breeders, are numerous, and of the Mussulmani faith.

Curriers, skinners, and shoemakers, are numerous, and chiefly cultivators, though some follow their trade, especially the last mentioned.

Water-carriers, are both Hindoo and Mussulmani: and the highest castes in Beekaneer drink from the mussŭk without hesitation.

There are a very few Hindwi gardeners.

There are a few Mussulmani cotton-cleaners.

There are a few Mussulmani butchers.

Hindwi scavengers, a few and only employed as such.

Dhers and Aheiries are very numerous. Mihturs are few in number. These low castes, can take horses to the Rajpoots, and are often employed as syces in this part of Rajwarra.

Of the religious devotee orders are gosains and soniyassies (some are atits) naths or jogies: there are also many jetties or jain priests: and byragies and sunjogies.

The hills are low, far apart, and few in number. Hills.

There are no rivers: and only a few small torrents in the Rivers. rains.

There are no lakes; tanks are however, numerous, both Lakes. natural and artificial; but none contain water beyond six months, even in the most favorable seasons.

Wells are rather numerous: the deepest are at Beekaneer Wells. and have a depth of 330 feet: the least deep in the principality have a depth of 120 feet. Some of the inhabitants pretend to have the power of indicating places where good water will be found; but are said generally to fail: these charlatans pretend to be guided by the smell of the earth. Occasionally good water is found; but, much more frequently it is bad. Some of the wells are very saline.

The inhabitants declare that some of the water has a poisonous quality: and that death even occurs a day subsequently to drinking it. They further say, that a cure is occasionally made, by cutting the ears deeply and allowing the blood to flow freely. This superstitious idea has probably arisen, owing to those exposed to the burning heat, being commonly attacked by determination of blood to the head, after being much overheated by travel, and on arriving at the well, drinking copiously of cold water: giving rise to apoplexy, when bleeding would of course relieve.

In digging the wells, the first 45 feet are of sand and then down to the water, of concrete rolled limestone (kunkul) in a silicious bed, or with argillaceous earth: chalk also occurs disaggregated (moorúr): yellow bole also occurs in deep beds, and is called (mêth or Mooltani mittie): the water is reached in variegated sandstone all over Beekaneer.

Bullocks and camels are used to draw the water: and another pair, are generally added to the rope, when the môt or skin of water is half way up.

Crops. There is no rubbee crop, except a very little near the canal on the borders of Hissar and Hansi. There is however generally a plentiful Khurreef crop, which consists chiefly of bujra and moth, and also of jowar and gowar phullie (not only as a vegetable, but as a grain). Turboozas, are very excellent, and occur both cultivated and wild. Kurboozas, kakris, moolies, piyaz, bhaingans, are cultivated by irrigation in the hot winds on a small scale.

Tax. The tax on cultivation is most unequally divided: the Rajpoot only pays $\frac{1}{10}$ in the 100: while the Jauts and others pay $\frac{1}{4}$ in the hundred, besides other exactions.

Manufactures. Some woollens of a finer kind are manufactured: and a great many of a coarser fabric, the wool of the sheep being superior: beautiful sugarcandy is also prepared, from imported goor.

Ores. Copper was formerly found. Impure limestone is abundant: also chalk, and yellow bole: red ochre is also abundantly found.

Salts. Saltpetre is made by collecting the saline matters mixed with dirt, from ths heaps of old bones and dung near the villages, after the rains. These sweepings are put in an earthen gurra, having a small hole in the bottom, and water is percolated through, and the solution is subsequently crystallized.

The camels are very fine and numerous : they are much Animals. prized : and are reared on the grass and "phog." A small sort of tiger (nahr) is found, with smooth head, yellow skin, and dark hairs mixed, with neither stripes nor spots (like the South American Jagouar ?). The fox, the jackal, the hyena, immense quantities of rats and mice, the wild hog, the hedgehog, the antilope ; the nylghau, the bear, are found wild. Horses are bred, and are sometimes superior. Donkeys and pariah dogs abound.

The birds are the peacock, the partridge (grey), the Birds. pigeon, the crow, the kite, the hawk, the sparrow, a sort of snipe, the parrot, and the bustard.

The common "maina" is said not to be found any where in Beekaneer.

Fish are not known to exist in the principality. Fish.

The serpents are, the cobra di capello (gohũna) : and Reptiles. two other varieties of coluber; the orange speckled kind (called goora) very numerous and fierce, and the black kind (or kurait) : another black speckled kind is also found (called parur) and is very numerous : the common boa constrictor attains a large size : and water-snakes are also found.

Scorpions and black ants are abundantly seen ; while the white ants (termites) are almost unknown : being only found on the very little black soil there is.

Grass is abundant; the species are chiefly sawan, dhoop, Grass. boorut (spear grass), ruchal, dab (poa cynosuroides), boor, sirkhunda, and gandhar, (khuss khuss, andropogon muricatum.)

Trees are very few and scattered : they are chiefly the Trees. bhoura or babool, the khejra, the jhal or peloo, the peepul, the burgud, the neem, the bukain, the rohira or reorha and the ak bush, and the phog every where : the wood of the latter is commonly burnt : the beir or berie also occurs both large and small*.

* Many of the plants and minerals of Rajpootanah, will be found arranged scientifically at the end of this Report.

Trade. A few roses, jasmines, and pomegranates are cultivated near Beekaneer in gardens.

Woolens and sugarcandy are exported. Many caravans pass from Sinde and Cabul on camels. There are very few brinjarras or bullock carriers.

Medicine. There are hakims, jetties, and bueds, who cannot be very good physicians, since the mild country intermittents are often allowed to remain two years.

Education. There was an English schoolmaster formerly entertained by the Raja. The brahmuns and jetties are the present teachers at Beekaneer: in the villages there are no oostàdjees at all.

Diseases. There is very little sickness usually at any season present in this principality. The fevers are few and mild, except when maltreated, are chiefly tertians, and attack during the rains. Dracunculus (guineaworm) is very common indeed. The sun frequently affects the head: and from this cause a good many deaths occur. The inhabitants generally are long-lived: even the eaters of opium and bhang: the two latter however become useless members of the society, becoming gradually listless and silly: they at length consume two tolas of opium per diem. Epilepsy is rather common: there are few insane. Small-pox is very severe and fatal. Hepatitis when it occurs is generally fatal. Cholera very seldom appears.

Seasons. The rains are very irregular; during this period thunder storms are very severe. In April, May and June, the heat of the weather is hardly bearable. In the cool season the thermometer is often very low, and ice commonly formed.

Soils. Soils generally sandy: sand and a little marl: concrete limestone and red sand: sand and a very little clay: and black loam in a very few places.

JESSULMEER.

Extent. Jessulmeer extends from the 26th to the 28th degree of north latitude, and from 70½ to the 73rd degree of east longitude: the extreme length is from near Girab north-eastward to Girrajsir, being 150 miles : and the extreme breadth is from Bap near Phulodee, north-west to the middle of the Great Desert about 78 miles.

The aborigines are Bhatties of the Yaduvansa Rajpoot division : and the Deora and Jessur Rajpoot tribes : the Oswal tribe of seths and bunyas : and Bheels now civilized in the villages :—and paliwal brahmuns in great numbers. Aborigines.

The present ruler is Raja Guj Singh, a Bhattie Rajpoot. Ruler.

The Rajpoots are chiefly Bhatties : there are also a good many of the Soda, Deora, Powar, Pahoo, and Jessur Rajpoot tribes. Tribes.

The brahmuns who conduct the worship, are of the Goozurgour tribe : the Palwŭl and Pokhurna brahmuns cultivate the soil.

The Oswal bunyas are a numerous and very wealthy body, this principality being considered by them as their fatherland.

The cultivators are in general all the poorest of whatsoever tribe.

The water-carriers are Hindoos, and convey the water on camels and *asses* : and all the highest castes even drink from these animals' burdens.

There is nothing else remarkable regarding the other divisions of inhabitants, which differ little from those of Beekaneer, previously spoken of.

There is one remarkable hill near Jessulmeer, of a fine grained yellow limestone, that has been applied to lithographic purposes : also a limestone breccia with a basis of red ochre, forms another smaller hill : there are also a few slight elevations sacttered over the country. Hills.

There are no rivers : and only a few torrents in the rains. Rivers.

There are no lakes ; but many tanks exist, both large and small : amongst which a few retain water all the year. By far the greater number dry up, and sometimes the whole. Lakes.

There are a few wells at the towns and villages : some contain pure water, while most are brackish, or even salt springs : nearly all are very deep : the deepest measure Wells.

450 feet: in a very few places water is near the surface. In digging sand is first passed through for many feet, and yellow bole earth, then sandstone, and the water is reached in a light yellow colored sandstone.

Cultivation. There is only a khurreef crop; but the bujra is very plentiful and excellent in quality: moong-ka-dal is also abundant and good: moth-ka-dal is here an inferior crop: the gowar-phullie is here also cultivated as a grain. The little wheat and grain sown in the cold season, yields in general a very inferior return: turboozas are wild and fine.

This principality is remarkable for producing very fine and large onions.

LandTax. The Raja receives only one-eighth from the ryots; so very poor is the soil.

FineArts. Very fine woollen shawls and cloth is made, the wool of the sheep being very superior: the best shawls cost 30 Rs.

Minerals. Saltpetre is made in small quantity.

Limestone has been exported for lithographic purposes.

Animals. The camels are very fine and numerous; an animal of the feline kind, similar to the Beekaneer one, is found: horses are bred of a superior kind and sell well elsewhere: the animals are otherwise the same as those in Beekaneer.

Vegetation. There are very few trees; though in some places the khejra is plentiful: the other trees that occur are similar to those of Beekaneer, only much less numerous. Grass is abundant, a few superior date trees grow near Jessulmeer.

Trade. A considerable trade in woollens, and a trifling trade in onions exists: lithographic stones were exported.

Medicine. The medicine is in the same state as in Beekaneer.

Education. Jetties and brahmuns teach the richer to read.

Diseases. The diseases are few in number, and even intermittent fever is by no means frequent in the rains. Guineaworm is a very common complaint. Small-pox is severe and fatal. Hepititis is rare. Cholera seldom visits this principality.

Opium is much eaten habitually, and does not seem to shorten life.

Seasons. The rains are very irregular: the cold is severe in the winter: the hot season is most oppressive.

Soils. The soil is chiefly sand; or, in many places, kunkul and sand with clay: and in the few gardens artificial soil.

Reptiles. The reptiles are nearly the same as in Beekaneer: one snake, however, called Peewanee is very poisonous; it is of a yellow colour, thick and short. Superstition. The superstitious natives say, that this snake does not bite; but, it comes (like incubus) during the night, and rests on the breast of the sleeper, and on leaving this situation strikes with its tail, and the person dies in the morning.

JODPOOR OR MARWAR.

Extent. Jodpoor extends from 24° 35′ to 27° 43′ north latitude: and from 70° 26′ to 75° 16′ east longitude: the greatest width is from Pokhurn or Phulodee, south eastwardly to the hills near Soojut, 150 miles: and the extreme length is from the mouth of the river Looni; north eastwardly to Ladnoo or to Marout, being 300 miles.

Aborigines. The aborigines may be first considered, as the race of Meenas, many of whom still inhabit Marwar, and the Bheel tribes both wild and civilized: the Jauts are however most numerous, and a very ancient race in this principality: there are also many Dhers and Aheiries; and after these the Purihar Rajpoots must be considered the most antique tribe: The very old town of Oosha in Marwar, is the original abode from whence the now numerous and immensely wealthy tribe of Oswal Seths and Bunyas have sprung: and this tribe though of the Jain sect, still among themselves feel pride in considering their Rajpoot descent.

The wild Bheels are a savage race; they are migratory, and are known by the name of "*Bhowries.*"

Ruler. The present ruler is Raja Maun Singh, Rhatore.

Tribes. The Rhatore tribe of Rajpoots is by far the most numerous: after this, the Bhattie, the Chohan, the Solankhie, the Purihar, the Manglia, and the Sankla tribes of Rajpoots are less numerous, as enumerated, in a decreasing ratio.

The priests who conduct the worship, are the Goozurgour and the Gour of the Ch ninayut tribe of brahmuns;

the Pokhurna brahmuns are very numerous, and both trade and cultivate.

The traders and merchants are chiefly Oswal, Maiserie, Suraogie, and Ugger-wallah tribes.

The cultivators are chiefly Jauts; but here as elsewhere all the poorer are so employed.

In this principality, there are a good many *Aheers* who are both cow-feeders and cultivators.

The water-carriers are of all castes, and convey the water on camels, bullocks, buffaloes or carts.

A tribe of "*Bhoois*" or bearers, is numerous, and the men are not only employed to carry burdens, but can prepare food for the Rhatore Raja and the Thakoors.

The begging tribes are very numerous, and the Naths partly govern and ruin the country.

The other tribes are much the same as those previously mentioned.

Hills. There are numerous hills scattered over the country, generally known by the name of "Bhom parbut;" i. e. hills of the soil: the small range on which Jodpoor and Mundore are built is designated by the name of those cities.

Rivers. The Looni, or salt river, runs into the Rin; its water is sweet as far as Balotra, beyond which town it becomes salt, and retains water flowing in a small stream all the year; but, above Balotra, the bed becomes dry after the rains. The Looni bounds the desert or "thul:" there are no other rivers; but, there are many torrents in the height of the rains.

Lakes. There are no lakes. Tanks are abundant in the towns and villages: some retain water all the year; but most dry up.

Wells. The wells are abundant, and in general from 30 to 90 feet in depth: the water is very generally good: in some places, as at Nagore, most of the wells become dry in the hot season; but in other places, as at Jodpoor, the wells generally retain abundance of water all the year. In digging the wells, sand is first passed through, then concrete lime (or kunkul), then hornblende schist, and the water is found in very hard granite, having numerous schorl crystals in it so as to be nearly black: the water when reached rises with rapidity even in the hot season.

By the aid of irrigation there is an abundant Rubbee crop: an inferior red and white wheat (called kuttea and pisooa) is produced abundantly: and in some dark alluvial deposits wheat grows without irrigation: barley is in general a plentiful crop: gram is sown where the soil suits it; but is not abundant. There is no sugar-cane cultivation. The Godwar district is the most fertile. Cultivation.

The Khurreef crop is also generally a very plentiful one: bujra and joar are very abundant; mukka is less so: moth ka dal is very abundant (the grain is used to feed horses, &c. as well as for food): til and moong ka dal are also often abundant crops: the gowar-phullie is here also cultivated as a grain.

The very few gardens are at the principal towns, and the anars produced at that barren spot, Jodpoor, are superexcellent.

A very small melon called "kachhari" grows abundantly wild and is very highly prized: also another kind called "khelera;" both are sent in presents to great distances.

The Raja receives in rent one-fifth of the produce. Land Tax.

Coarse woollens, chiefly red in colour, are manufactured. Ivory articles are made at Jodpoor; where also the gold and silver work is superior. Swords and matchlocks are well made. Coloured play-things are made at, and even exported from, Jodpoor.—So poor is the state of the arts in Marwar! Arts.

Salt is abundantly produced at Sambhur, Punchbudra, Deedwanah, Phulodee, and the Looni river. Fine calcareous alabaster and white marble abound at Mukrani, Fine grained light yellow sandstone at Khator. Iron ore is also found in some places. Minerals.

The camels are fine and plentiful: bullocks are very fine, from the Jhalore and Nagore districts: horses are superior from the Mewar and Talore districts: sheep and goats are very abundant: the dark yellow sort of tiger with- Animals.

out stripes is also found in this principality: the lion (called nahr-singh) is found in the Godwar district: where also the royal tiger and ounce abound: wild hogs are numerous.

The other animals are much the same as those previously mentioned.

Vegetation. Jungles, with and without trees, abound: in some parts of the principality trees are plentiful: the khejra (mimosa edibilis) is most abundant: then the babool: the burgud and peepul near towns: the jhal or peeloo: the kurēla: various acacias: the bier or ber both large and small: the rohira in sandy moist situations: the neem in plenty: grass is abundant: phog is not common: khunsera (eaten by camels) is plentiful: the ak or madar is large and very common, (used even in building the roofs of the houses:) the bukain and jeyt are abundant near cultivation: and sissoo, though very scarce, is of excellent dark quality.

Trade. A very great carrying trade, viâ Pali, from Sinde, Cashmeer, Cabul, Bombay, and Delhi exists at present, and has so existed for ages. Camels, horses, and bullocks are exported, some horses sell for 700 Rs.: grain is exported: ivory articles, dyed leather and petarrahs are exported from Jodpoor: iron utensils from Nagore: and a substance called "koomkum," made of turmeric and lime juice, is made and exported to great distances, being used for the "teeka" on the forehead at marriages.

Medicine. In the same way, as in other parts of Rajwarra, the Jetties conduct the medical and surgical treatment, aided in the latter by the "*baburs*" who are "*surgeons*" by caste and occupation.

Education. At Jodpoor there is a considerable Poshal, or school, supported by the Raja; there is said also to be one in every large town: the state of education is, however, lamentable.

Diseases. The climate is generally healthy, fevers of all types are common in the rains, but are seldom severe: cholera is sometimes very severe: "the plague" was very fatal at Jodpoor, Nagore, Pali and Mairta: dysentery is not uncommon: colics are very frequent: guineaworm is very common: hemorrhoids very frequent, from the abuse of opium. Opium eating is very prevalent, and does not shorten life; but those who abuse it become useless to themselves and others.

The rains are very irregular: the hot season is severe: the cool season often very cold, and ice is frequently spontaneously formed. In April and May rain occasionally falls, in some years, and then bujra is sown, and lives till the regular rains set in, and forms a very heavy crop. Seasons.

Soils chiefly sand: black soil in some places, especially in Godwar: white earth (dhobe mittie) being marl with sand, is a very common soil. Soils.

The reptiles do not differ from those of Beekaneer, except that the Peewana snake does not occur in Marwar. Reptiles.

JAEPOOR.

Jaepoor extends from 25° 50′ to 27° 50′ north latitude, and from 74° 40′ to 77° 20′ east longitude; being 120 miles from north to south, measuring from near the town of Gowrie to the Sabee-nuddee: and 160 miles from east to west, measuring from Kunwye Larkani, to beyond Sarout. Extent.

Meenas were the aboriginal inhabitants, and their capital was Amber before they were conquered by the Cuchwaha Rajpoots: to this day these Meenas are a numerous race, and unlike the generality of Meenas have remained unmixed Hindoos: some tribes of Bheels were also aboriginal. Aborigines.

Ruler. Raja Siwaie Ram Singh, Cuchwaha; he is now only six years of age, and the country is governed by a regency: the Majee and the regency are at present great enemies: and the country is in a very disorganized state. Ruler.

The Rajpoots are chiefly of the Cuchwaha tribe: a few of the other Rajpoot tribes are scattered about. Tribes.

The Chinnayut tribe of brahmuns performs all the priestly offices of the Rajpoots and other high castes: the Bagrie brahmuns are of very ancient date, and conduct the worship of the Meenas: also many others of different Gowtries are at Jaepoor and other towns.

The cultivators are chiefly Meenas: the Jauts are also a numerous race: and next to these the Cuchwaha Rajpoots, and all the poorer classes in the villages, whether of high or low caste: amongst the latter are many Aheiries, Dhers, &c.

The water-carriers are Hindoos and Mussulmans, and convey the water on bullocks or camels; but here water is not conveyed upon asses.

A sort of Hindoo surgeons called "Baburs" are common at Jaepoor and in other towns; they chiefly confine their business to surgery of a rude kind; but, also sometimes act as barbers: a few of these people are scattered over Rajwarra.

Common barbers, or naies are numerous; they not only shave and attend to the persons of their employers; but can, and often do, dress the rich Rajpoots' victuals.

The Nagas (or naked Byragies) are a numerous body; they are supported by jaghires from the state: and serve as sepahies in their own regiments: they do not now go naked: they are a very unruly useless body of men.

The other tribes are not in any way remarkable.

Hills. A part of the Aravulli range of hills extends to Rintimbore. On the Amber hills, the cities of Jaepoor and Amber are placed. The Tora hills extend near Rajmahl, on the Bunas. The Malkhet hills are in Shekawattie. The Byranie hills, and other small ranges are scattered over the country, which is, however, generally level.

Rivers. The Bunas is a large river, and rises from beyond Saimul, in Mewar, in the Aravulli range: it is joined by the Beris from Oodipoor, and many other streams, and after a long and tortuous course joins the Chumbul at the holy "sungum" of Rameswar; forcing its way through "Sat-parra" (or seven distinct ranges). The Bhandie is a small river which flows all the year. The Sirsootie-nuddee, close to Jaepoor, flows all the year. The Bhan-gunga, is a wide stream or rather torrent in the heavy rains, nearly a mile across: but rapidly becomes a dry bed again. The Thantra ka nuddee flows all the year. And there is an immense number of rain torrents.

Wells. The wells are very abundant, most are from 15 to 30

feet in depth: some are even 75 feet deep: though in some wells the water is brackish the generality contain pure water. Water is very abundant, and near the surface, especially between Ajmeer and Jaepoor. In digging the wells sand or sandy loam is commonly met with: in many places the well wall (or cylinder of masonry) is first erected, and then is sunk in by excavation. The water is, however, sometimes reached in schistose rock, granite, or sandstone.

The Rubbee crop, by the aid of plenty of manure and abundant irrigation, is in general very plentiful: barley and wheat are chiefly produced: also mustard, the poppy (for opium), the coriander, and carroway seed: in the black alluvial deposits near rivers and the beds of talaos, grain grows well, and is as elsewhere, never irrigated. Cultivation.

The Khurreef crop is still more abundant: bujra, joar, mukka (Indian corn) being produced in great quantities: moong ka dal, moth ka dal, and til are also in plenty, some rice is grown in a few favorable situations: and sugar-cane on a small scale. The ryots are much depressed.

The gardens at Jaepoor and other large towns are fine, and abound in vegetables and fruits.

The architecture of Jaepoor (which is the finest city in India), is very superior; part of the interior of the palace is superb and imposing, and altogether has given a justly great celebrity to the name of Raja Jae Singh the founder. Painting and the general arts are in a more advanced state, than elsewhere in Rajwarra. The shoes of Jaepoor are famous, and are exported in large quantities to Sinde and elsewhere. The dying and brass work are superior. Sculpture is also practised, in the formation of small marble images, that sell for considerable sums. FineArts.

A good deal of copper is procured in Shekawattie: abundance of iron is found, marble in some places: common limestone and concrete limestone in plenty: sandstone and mica and hornblende schist in abundance: marl (called pandoo or pandol mittie) is in immense beds, very common below the surface, especially about Doodoo: salt from the Sambhur lake and soil; saltpetre is also extracted. Minerals.

Animals. The camels are numerous and good; but are not so superior as those of Beekaneer or Marwar: the bullocks are inferior: horses are bred and some are fine: tigers are numerous in the wooded hills: the lion is said to be found: leopards, panthers and ounces are plentiful: there are many kinds of deer, and most of the animals commonly found in jungles.

Vegetation. There is almost every where abundance of grass: the hills are mostly covered with the large and small "dhao" trees: the khejra is very abundant, and when old is a good wood: the babool, kheir, peepul, peepur, burgud, neem, bukain, jhal or peeloo, rohira, sissoo, bier, gondie, furash, jhao, dhawra, jeyt, khujoor, khunsera, ak or madar, &c., are all more or less abundant.

Trade. Numerous caravans pass through from Rewarree and many other places; brass vessels, coloured coarse cottons, plain coarse cotton, shoes, and fruits (jujubes and oranges) are exported, and a few small sculptured articles.

Medicine. Medicine is in the same state as elsewhere in Rajwarra.

Education. The same may be said regarding the state of education.

Diseases. This principality is sometimes very healthy, and at others is very much the reverse. Fevers are very common in the rains: cholera is severe at long intervals: guineaworm is much less common than in Marwar: dysentery is not prevalent: opium is much eaten, especially by the Rajpoots and Meenas, who often become quite useless from this indulgence; but the inhabitants declare life is not shortened by its use.

Seasons. The seasons are irregular, especially the rains: the climate is very oppressive in the hot season, and very cold in the winter.

Soils. The eastern and southern portions of this principality are chiefly a very light loamy soil of a red colour, and in some parts a deep black loam: the western is nearly pure sand: near Jaepoor, a light yellow loam is found beneath the sand: the northern is sand, and in some places a little brown loamy soil: whitish marly soil (khattie or dhobe mittie) is found at Doodoo and elsewhere: in some parts "kunkuli" soil occurs, and is very barren.

Reptiles—A small white whip snake with black stripes is found in this principality, which if pursued can leap several yards clear off the ground. The other reptiles are the same as elsewhere.

MEWAR.

Mewar extends 24° 15′ to 26° 10′ north latitude: and from 72° 55′ to 75° 45′ east longitude; being in extreme length north and south 115 miles: and in extreme breadth, east and west 117 miles. Extent.

This is a very fertile region, presenting every variety of surface, and is known as the garden of Rajwarra. It is the most ancient of the present Rajpoot principalities.

The aborigines are Bheels of the old pure or "Oojla" stock; now chiefly known as "Bhoomia Bheels," descended from a mixture of the "Solanki" Rajpoot with the "Oojla" Bheel. Aborigines.

After the massacre of the ancestors of the Ranas of Mewar, when they were expelled from Guzerat (or Saurashtra), one of the queens, by name Pooshpavati, escaped and found refuge amongst some brahmun inhabitants of the Mallia mountains: the queen was delivered of a son in a cave of these hills, from which circumstance she called him Goha (or cave born): and hence arose one of the designations of the Rana's tribe "Gehlote." Goha subsequently associated with the Bheels, and was on one occasion, in sport, elected as their sovereign, when a young Bheel chief having accidently cut his thumb applied the blood to Goha's forehead, as the "teeka" of investiture. However simple the origin, this practice is still kept up at the court of Oodipoor: and on every investiture of the Ranas of Mewar, the Oguna Bheel chief, makes the bloody teeka on his sovereign's forehead, drawing the blood from a small incision in the thumb, after which he takes the prince by the arm and seats him on the throne: the Oondree Bheel chief holds the salver of spices and sacred grains of rice on the same occasion.

Ruler. Ruler. Rana Sirdar Singh: Gehlote or Sesodiya; is the most noble of the 36 Sachæ or royal Rajpoot tribes: directly descended from Loh, the eldest son of Rama. The tribe first founded or conquered Lohore or Lohkote; and when driven thence, the Gehlotes conquered and governed Guzerat or Saurashtra, until, again expelled, they found refuge (as before stated) in Mewar. The Ranas are of the elder branch of the Suriya-vansa, or children of the sun. The Hindoo tribes unanimously acknowledge the Rana's claim as the representative of Rama, under the name of "Hindooa Sooruj," or Sun of the Hindoos.

Tribes. The principal tribe of Rajpoots now inhabiting is the Sesodiya, and is also the most numerous: a good many of the other Rajpoot tribes are also scattered over the country.

There are many tribes of brahmuns; but at Nathdwarra the Diva brahmuns are most numerous, as the worshippers of Krishna. Many brahmuns are also cultivators.

The followers of Jin or Jain are a numerous and wealthy body in Mewar: and their Jetties or priests have very considerable influence.

The cultivators are of many tribes; but chiefly are Jauts, Bheels, Rajpoots and brahmuns. The Jauts were wisely introduced from Marwar by one of the Ranas.

Charuns and Bhats are a numerous body in Mewar.

The other tribes are of the same castes as those in other parts of Rajwarra:—amongst which, however, the naie or barber (though of very low caste) is a favoured individual, as he can be employed to prepare the food of the Rana and other Sesodiya chiefs.

Hills. The surface of Oodipoor is very generally hilly: abounding in many scattered low ranges. The chief range, varying in height from 100 to 4000 feet above the base, is the Aravulli, which extends from the south-west of Mount Aboo, nearly as far as Delhi, though under different appellations.

Rivers. The chief river, in relation to the length of its course, is the Bunas, already mentioned; but the Chumbul, although only flowing a short distance through Mewar (near Byusrore) deserves chief mention, from the considerable magnitude.

The Chumbul rises from the northern side of the most elevated part of the Vindhya range of mountains in Malwa : the Chumbul is joined by the Sepra, Peepuldeo, and Chota Sinde, the Kali Sinde, the Sodura, the Newuz and the Parbuttie on the right side ; and by the Bunas on the left. The Chumbul enters Mewar near Shamgurh, and is there a very considerable stream : the length of *his* course is about 500 miles : and along his banks specimens of almost every race now in India may be found.

The Beris is a minor river, and joins the Bunas.

Small streams and rain torrents are numerous in every direction.

There are no natural lakes in Mewar ; but, the semi-natural lakes are very extensive, and magnificent at Oodipoor. Tanks are abundant all over Mewar, and in general retain water all the year. Lakes.

The wells are plentiful, and the water is in general near the surface : many contain brackish water, and a sweet well and a brackish one are often in vicinity. Wells.

The cultivation is of every variety : from the finest sugarcane to the commonest "Kodo" rice : the poppy is much cultivated : the crops are generally excellent. Cultivation.

Almost the only manufactures are of coarse cotton cloths, and of matchlocks and swords. Arts.

The Aravulli and many other hills, being of primary formation, render it very probable that many metallic veins might be found. Rich mines are said formerly to have existed. The mines were and still are royalties ; their produce increasing the revenue of the prince. As a proof that metals must formerly have been more plentifully extracted, and of considerable value, the sovereign rights of "An," "Dan," "Kan," may be mentioned, which have been asserted from time immemorial ; the meaning of the words being "allegiance, commercial duties, and mines." The tin mines of Mewar are recorded to have been once very productive, and are said also to have yielded silver : Minerals.

these mines are not now worked. Copper is abundant and supplies the currency. Sulphuret of Antimony is also found. Iron is very plentiful.

Some inferior precious stones have been found.

A scientific examination of the hills of Mewar, would probably lead to important results.

Animals. Every kind of animal common in India is found, (excepting the wild elephant and rhinoceros :) horses and camels are bred of a good quality.

Vegetation. Vegetation is in general abundant, and in some places luxuriant. An immense variety of forest trees ornaments the jungles.

Trade. Grain is exported in large quantities in favourable seasons : opium is largely exported : coarse cotton cloths and arms are also exported.

Medicine. Medicine is chiefly in the hands of the Jetties : and in the same state as elsewhere in Rajwarra.

Education. Education is under the superintendence of the brahmuns and Jetties.

Diseases. Epidemics are rather frequent: cholera, when it appears, is generally severe : fevers are very common during and after the rains, and often of a remittent type and fatal : the plague carried off thousands at Bednore, Bhilwarra and other places : small-pox is fatal and common in the hot season : guineaworm is not very common : opium is much eaten by the Rajpoots and other tribes.

Seasons. The seasons are more regular than in the northern parts of Rajwarra : the rains are generally abundant.

Soils. The soil is very generally of a light loam; but every variety of soil is met with.

Reptiles. The snakes are of the kinds usually met with.

KOTAH.

Extent. Kotah forms by far the larger division of Harowtee, or Haravati : it is irregular in figure, and extends from 23° 45′ to 25° 50′ north latitude : and from 75° 35′ to 70° 30′ of east longitude; being in extreme length from north to south 125 miles: and in extreme breadth from east to west 115 miles.

The aboriginal inhabitants were the Oojula Bheels, and the Bhoomia Bheels, and Meenas: all of which tribes are still very numerous. Aborigines.

The Rajpoots are chiefly of the Hara tribe: many others of the different Rajpoot tribes are also inhabitants.

The present rule is divided between Maha Rao Ram Singh; who governs two thirds of the country separately; he is of the ancient race of princes and a Hara Rajpoot: and Maha Raja Mudhun Singh, who has one-third of the country distinctly under his control: he is of the Jhala Rajpoot tribe, and is the descendant of the famous Zalim Singh, the celebrated minister of Kotah, who so long ruled his master and the state also, kept out the Maharattas, and aided and courted the British amidst apparently great difficulties. Ruler.

The great body of cultivators are Meenas, Bheels and Goozurs: all the poorer tribes however, without relation to caste, also cultivate here as elsewhere. Tribes.

The hills are not very numerous in Kotah; one extensive range, the "Durra," runs from beyond Girdhurpoor to Shêrgurh, and nearly in the centre is situated the famous Mookundurra ghaut: other hills are scattered in various points; but the country is in general flat. Hills.

The Chumbul separates Kotah from Boondee: the Kali-Sinde and the Newuz, water the soil: and a great number of nuddees, retaining water all the year, are every where met with, excepting amongst the hills. Rivers.

There are no natural lakes; but artificial tanks are very plentiful, and retain abundance of water all the year. Lakes.

Wells are every where abundant, and the water is near the surface. In digging wells, black loam is first passed through, then at a certain depth a stiff yellow clay is found, in which water is met with; but near the banks of the Chumbul, sandstone more or less thick has to be penetrated, and after cutting through about 15 feet, water appears in the soil found below the stone: about Kotah, quartz Wells.

rock is also very common, or quartz with hornblende and schorl.

Cultivation. The crops, both Rubbee and Khurreef, are excellent: wheat is universally cultivated and used of three kinds; the julalea (a beautiful, large, white-grained wheat), the kutea, and the pisea: barley is not sown: the poppy is very largely cultivated: and this practice has much injured the country: sugar-cane for which the soil is peculiarly favourable, though still cultivated, is very much neglected: rice is much cultivated, wherever plenty of water can be commanded, so as to flood the ground. Almost every species of agricultural produce that is grown elsewhere, is cultivated here.

The gardens are very fine and productive, especially near the city of Kotah.

Arts. Fine coloured cotton cloths: coarse cotton cloths, and brass vessels, are manufactured of a superior kind.

Minerals. Copper ore was formerly worked near Dhunwarra; but is not extracted now; iron is still produced, but not in great plenty; soft sandstone abounds: also kunkul and other concrete lime-stone, used to make lime: marble is said to be found amongst the hills.

Vegetation. Vegetation is very luxuriant; almost every kind of forest tree and shrub is found in the extensive forests in the hilly parts and near the Chumbul, and amongst others the teak tree is not uncommon.

Trade. There is a great trade in grain in favourable seasons: vast quantities of opium are exported: fine and coarse cottons, and brass vessels are exported: great numbers of brinjarras annually pass.

Medicine. Medicine is as unscientific as elsewhere in Rajwarra.

Education. Education is in the hands of the Chuinayut brahmuns. An English teacher has been obliged to leave, owing to want of encouragement.

Diseases. Harowtee is very unhealthy, especially near the city of Kotah: the jungles are fatally dangerous for a great part of the year: strangers, on arrival, are very liable to attacks of remittent fevers: cholera is very frequent and severe, and

Animals. Tigers are abundant: bears also: all kinds of deer: camels are excellent for loading and in great plenty: horses are bred: the breed of cattle is small, but plenty: all sorts of game abound almost certainly recurs, every second or third year. In all Harowtee, guineaworm is very frequent: and is most troublesome in the rains. Rheumatism is very common. Opium is much eaten.

The rains are regular, and the climate is then very damp: the hot season is very oppressive: the cold months are in general agreeably pleasant. Seasons.

The soil is generally a rich black loam: other lighter soils are sometimes met with: where the stiff yellow loam comes to the surface, good crops are not produced. The wheat is never irrigated here. The poppy is, however, very carefully watered. Soils.

The common venomous snakes are found: and in the hills the boa constrictor attains a very great size. Reptiles.

BOONDEE.

Boondee extends from 25° 10′ to 25° 55′ of north latitude; and from 75° 12′ to 76° 25′ of east longitude; being in length from north to south 45 miles, and in breadth from east to west, 73 miles. Extent.

Meenas were chiefly the aboriginal tribe. Bheels also are a very ancient race here: both are still numerous: the Boondee Bheels are distinguished into the "Oojula," who only eat the flesh of killed animals: and the "Mila" who eat carrion. Aborigines.

The present prince is Maha Rao Ram Singh, a Hara Rajpoot. Ruler.

The Rajpoots are chiefly of the Hara tribe: other Rajpoot tribes are scattered over the country. Tribes.

The other different castes are of the same tribes as those enumerated under the head of Kotah.

The Boondee hills are extensive, and form a principal pass at the city itself, into the Mewar and the Ajmeer states; smaller ranges are scattered in many places, and one rather extensive range is near to Naogong. Hills.

The Chumbul divides Boondee from Kotah: the Tolera nuddee retains water, in some places, all the year: as does also the Ghora-puchar, more or less, and is a torrent dan- Rivers.

gerous (as the name implies) to horsemen in the rains: torrents are abundant during the rains.

Lakes. There are no natural lakes; but artificial talaos are plentiful near the larger towns, and retain water all the year.

Wells. The wells are numerous, and the water is generally near the surface; but at Boondee city is at a depth of 60 or 70 feet. The water is almost every where fresh.

Cultivation. Both the Rubbee and the Khurreef crops are excellent; wheat is generally cultivated, in the black soil without irrigation, and in the lighter soils it is watered: barley is cultivated to the north, where the soil nearly assimilates that of Ajmeer. The poppy is less cultivated than in Kotah. The sugar-cane is much cultivated about Naogong: it is of the smallest kind and is not watered.

Arts. Arms of various kinds are well made: other arts are not pursued with better success than is common elsewhere.

Minerals. Iron ore is abundant and yields good iron; as the hills are of primitive character, various metallic oxides are probably contained. Coarse marble is plentiful.

Animals. Animals are found of the same kind as those of Kotah, excepting the camels, which are superior.

Vegetation. The same plants are found as in Kotah; the vegetation is, however, much less luxuriant.

Trade. Iron is exported; also grain and sugar in favourable seasons. Large caravans frequently pass through, paying duty to the Rajah.

Diseases. The diseases are similar to those of Kotah: the climate is, however, on the whole less unhealthy.

Seasons. The seasons differ little from what is experienced at Kotah.

Soils. The soil is generally fertile and black; but becomes lighter and more sandy towards the northern parts.

Reptiles. Venomous snakes are more plentiful than those of Kotah.

SIROHIE.

Sirohie is a small principality to the westward of Marwar, to which state Sirohie is feudatory. The Jodpoor legion is stationed in Sirohie, and has a medical officer attached. It would therefore seem presumption in me, were I to allude to the medical topography.

MAIRWARRA.

Mairwarra is in that portion of the Aravulli chain between Komulmēr and Ajmeer, a space of about 90 miles in length, and varying in width from 6 to 20 miles. This country is surrounded and intersected in every direction by hills, which to the south-west rise to very considerable elevations. The "Mer" or "Mera" is the hill-man of this part of Rajpootanah, and Mairwarra means the region of hills. The term "Mer," applied to the inhabitants, is local; as they are in reality only a branch of the "Meenas" or "Mainas," one of the aborigines of India. Bounds.

The "Mers" are a sub-branch of the "Cheetas" who are an important division of the "Meenas." Aborigines.

These "Cheeta Meenas" claim connexion with the last of the "Chohan" emperors of Delhi, through his grandson Unail, who was descended from the Chohan king by a "Meena" concubine, and who became a voluntary exile from Ajmeer and associated with the wild "Meena" tribes; by his "Meena" wife he had a son called Cheeta, from whom the present "Cheetas" are descended. These are the men in power now in Mairwarra. The descendants of Cheeta, who occupied the northern frontier near Ajmeer, became Mahommedans, early in the reign of the Mogul emperors of Delhi, and Doodoh their chief, was named Dawud Khan by the hakim of Ajmeer, and created "Khan of Athoon," the place of his residence, and was then chief of all Mairwarra.

Anoop, another descendant of the Chohan king of Delhi, also married a "Meena" woman, by whom he had Burrar, whose descendants are still true to their original faith.

The "Mers" are divided into the Mahommedan sect, and those of the original tenets.

These people have always been notorious for lawless habits, In 1821 the "Mers" and "Cheetas" succumbed, without fighting, to the three corps sent against them.

The Mairwarra Local Battalion was subsequently raised, and is composed chiefly of "Mers;" it is a very fine corps; the Head Quarters are at Beawr. The district, under the superintendence of Captain Dixon, has been wonderfully improved, and is still improving.

Mers marry Widows.

The "Mers" (and also one or two ancient brahminical and Rajpoot tribes) have no objection to marrying widows: on such occasions amongst the "Mers," the bridegroom twines peepul leaves, instead of palm leaves, into his nuptial turban: in marrying a virgin palm leaves only are used. Many of their customs are according to the Hindoo ritual: such as the "sat-pheera," or seven perambulations round the "gurras" piled up and filled with grain: the "gat-jora" or uniting the garments: and the "hathleva" or junction of hands by the bride and bridegroom.

Curious Customs.

The Mahommedan "Mers" are still married by brahmuns.

If a "Mer" desires to divorce his wife, he gives her a shred of his turban, and places two gurras of water on her head, and sends her off: any one taking off the two gurras may claim the woman. This practice is called "jehar-le-nikala:" the same ceremony is also used by "Meenas," "Jauts," "Goozurs," "Aheers," and "Mallees."

The "Cheeta" or northern "Mer" swears by Allah, or by Doodoh Dawud Khan, or "Cheeta Burrar Khan." The southern "Mers" swear also by the last oath, and by "Sooruj ka sogun" and Natha ka sogun.

The Mahommedan "Mers" will not now eat hog. The southern "Mers" refuse nothing as food: and only respect the cow, out of regard to the "Nathas" or "Jogis" who have become their spiritual guides.

The district under Captain Dixon, is about 40 coss long, by 15 coss wide. The remainder of Mairwarra is subjected to the Rana of Oodipoor.

As a medical officer is stationed at Beawr, it would be superfluous in me to speak of the medical topography.

AJMEER.

The district of Ajmeer extends from 25° 35′ to 26° 40′ north latitude; and from 74° 25′ to 75° 27′ 30″ east longitude; being in length 65 miles, and in breadth 62½ miles. The town and district of Shapoora, to the south of Ajmeer is a dependency. Extent.

The first possessors of the soil and hills of this province were "Meenas," "Mers," and "Bheels;" but at a very early period these were subjected to conquerors, and by degrees almost suppressed: so that now a few "Meenas" only are to be found, and hardly a "Bheel" is to be met with: and the "Mers" are congregated in their own Mugra or hilly region. Aborigines.

At the earliest periods, Ajmeer, then not so called, was taken possession of by the "Purihar" Rajpoot princes of Mundore, who ruled extensively in the period of their glory: the present district, at that time formed only a very small part of the "Purihar" raja's possessions in Rajwarra. Purihara Rajpoots.

The "Purihara" is one of the four "Aguicula" tribes; races who obtained a footing in India, posteriorly to the "Suriyas" (or sun-descended) and the "Indus" (or moon-descended) Rajpoots. They claim Cashmeer as the country whence they migrated into India.

The Aguiculas are the Pramara, the "Purihara," the "Solanki," and the "Chohan."

Tradition pretends that they were created by the brahmuns to defend the altars of Iswarra (the Supreme Being) against the attacks of the "dytes" or atheists. They are believed to have been formed, by the aid of fire, on Mount Aboo: and the contests between these four creations and the ministers of the sun are said to have been fought there. Agnicula History.

The "Aguicoonda" is still shewn on Mount Aboo, where the miraculous creation is supposed to have taken place. The learned pundits explain the fable by supposing that the four warlike races were induced by the brahmuns to fight in defence of Hindoo polytheism, against the Buddhists and other deists, who must at that time have been very numerous, as the many remains of their temples prove.

Pramara. The Pramara (meaning chief warrior) was the most powerful race of the "Agniculas:" and consisted of 35 "Sachæ" or branches. There is still an old proverb "that the world is the Pramaras:" and the "No-kote-maroosth-ulli" signified the nine divisions into which the country from the Sutledge to the ocean was divided amongst them.

Raja Ram, Pramar, held his court at Tellingana in the Dukhan, and is recorded as universal sovereign of India.

At present, no vestige of independence exists to mark the greatness of the "Pramaras:" the only records of their power are ruins. The prince of Dhat in the Indian desert, whose adherents are known as the "Soda" tribe of Rajpoots, is the last phantom of royalty of this race, and he is a tributary. The Soda Rajpoots are supposed to be the same as the "Sogdi" mentioned by Arrian.

Chohan The "Chohan" or "Chahuman" is supposed to be the most valiant of the races of the "Agnicula" and perhaps of the whole Rajpoot race; owing to the tradition that the "Chohans" succeeded in subduing the "dytes" when the other Agniculas had failed. This race has always been the foremost in arms. It is divided into 24 Sachæ; and of these, the "Haras," the "Kheechees," the "Deoras," and the "Sonigurras," still maintain their names.

The "Chohans" count twenty-nine princes, from Anhul, the first created "Chohan," down to Pirthi Raj, the last Hindoo emperor of Delhi.

At present the most celebrated of this race, are the ruling families (Haras) of Boondee and Kotah: after them the "Kheechees" of Gagrown, the "Deoras" of Sirohie, and the "Soni gurras" of Jhalore.

Solankhie. The "Solankhie" is divided into sixteen branches scattered now over Rajwarra; they are also called "Chalook," and are the third Agnicula race, and are stated to have become rulers at Sooru on the Ganges before the "Rahtores" obtained Canouj. Their tribes inhabited Mooltan in the eighth century, and also are said to have ruled at Callian in Malabar. One of their princes, deposing the "Chohan" raja of Anhulwarra, ruled there at the time of the invasion of that place by Mahmood of Ghuzni.

The chief of Roopnagurh in Mewar is a "Solankhie:" and there are many petty chiefs of this tribe in Guzerat.

The "Purihara" or "Prithwihara" is the fourth and least of the "Agniculas:" they were early conquered by and in subjection to the "Tuars" of Delhi and the "Chohans" of Ajmeer. Purihara.

They were once, however, a great people: Mundore was their capital, and was the chief city of Marwar at that time, when the whole province owned the sway of this tribe, previous to the invasion of the "Rhatores," whose emigrant princes found an asylum with the "Purihar" Rana, when obliged to fly from Canouj; and subsequently Choudas, the "Rhatore," treacherously dispossessed the last of the "Purihar" princes.

The "Rawul" of Mewar first assumed the title of "Rana" from the Purihar, on the occasion of taking (with his "Gehlotes") Mundore, by storm.

The "Purihar" race is now few in numbers, and scattered over the face of Rajwarra. No independent chieftainship exists. At the confluence of the Cohari, the Sinde and the Chumbul, a small colony of "Puriharas" is located; being all that remains of a powerful race, once divided into twelve "sachæ."

The last of the "Purihar" monarchs was Nahur Rao, whose tomb is still extant at Mundore.

Aja Pal, the first "Chohan" Raja of Ajmeer, was said to have been, as his name implies, a goatherd, whose piety in daily supplying a saint at Poshkur with goat's milk, procured him a territory from the "Purihar" Rana. On the Nag-puhar, or serpent rocks, (a line of steep hills, two miles west of the Ana-sagur lake of Ajmeer,) in the middle of which is the pass to Poshkur, was the scene of Aja Pal's early days, and satisfied with that spot, he commenced building a fortress there, the extensive and massy walls of which are still visible: evidently constructed at a very remote Aja Pal.

period to defend the pass; the tradition states that his evil genius knocked down during the night what was built during the day: and therefore Aja Pal abandoned the spot, and went over to the opposite range, three miles eastward, and in time constructed the celebrated fort, called after him Aja-meer, on the highest summit; which, previously to being named Aja-meer (or Aja's hill), appears to have been named Gurh Beetli from a fort of the "Purihar" Ranas placed on it: the present name of Taragurh, was given after the great additions made to it by the Mahommedans.

Raos of Ajmeer.

At a much less remote time, so powerful were the "Chohans" of Ajmeer, that the princes of Cheetore, and Udiya Dit the chief of the "Pramaras" (who is said to have lived A. D. 1096) both served under the "Rao" of Ajmeer.

The proselytizing Mahommedans, under a general of the Caliph Walid the conqueror, are said to have been the first of the creed who visited India, and are stated to have penetrated from the Delta of the Indus, as far as (Ajmeer, A. D. 680), and to have sacked the place and returned as they came.

From Aja Pal, the shepherd king, Manika Raie is the principal person in the list of "Raos," down to the famed Beesila-deva or Vis-ala-deva.

Manika Raie.

Manika Raie was killed in the first century of the "Hijra," fighting against the Mahommedan general, Roshun Ally; whose army, viâ Sinde and Anjar, on the sea coast, came to attack Ajmeer, A. D. 722. After Manika Raie was slain, his son Lot, the heir apparent, was pierced by an arrow of a follower of Roshun Ally's, while standing on one of the battlements of the fort: and hence Lot is now one of the principal "Kool-devas" or penates of the "Chohans." These were the first Rajpoots of eminence slain by the Mahommedans.

Lot

Beesila-deva.

After many intermediate princes, Beesila-deva succeeded to the throne of Ajmeer, and headed a confederacy of the Hindoo kings, chased the descendants of Mahmood from Hindusthan, and ultimately obtained the "Chukur burthi" or universal dominion of India.

According to Colonel Todd, the victories gained were the origin of the recording column of iron, now seen at the Cootub minar near Delhi. Recorded on a column of Iron at Delhi.

This sovereign excavated the Beesila-talao of Ajmeer.

The third in succession to Beesila-deva was Ana Rao, a peaceful prince, who formed the Ana-sagur at Ajmeer.

Some generations after the demise of Ana Rao, Prithwi Rao succeeded, who also obtained, and was the last "Chohan" who held universal dominion, his real name was Peethora; but, when he obtained the "Chukur burthi" he changed his name to Prithwi; or the universe. Ana Rao.

Prithwi Rao, after many repulses by the Mahommedans, was at length attacked at Ajmeer by the Mahommedan general Allah-ood-deen, on the latter invasion under Mahmood of Ghuzni, who came, viâ Delhi, defeated Prithwi Rao, and took him away prisoner, A. D. 1015. After which he soon died. Prithwi Rao.

Allah-ood-deen left Meera Saheb as the hakim of Ajmeer. Meera Saheb.

Soon after the "Chohans" of the province rose and took the fort by surprise (or chappai sai); but, soon abandoned it again.

The Mahommedan power at Ajmeer ceased from the time of the defeat of Mahomed Shah at Delhi by Nadir Shah, A. D. 1745.

The "Rhatores" then came in and seized Ajmeer and the surrounding districts. Rhatores.

The "Rhatores" were driven out by the "Maharattas" in 1749, under their leader Apa Singh: and the "Maharattas" held possession till the British received the cession from Scindiah in 1818; when the "Maharatta" troops in the fort still held out; but, on demonstrations of attack being made, they gave in on promise of payment of their arrears. Maharattas.

Since that period, Ajmeer has been a British district. British.

The Ajmeer district is divided into ten purgunahs: these are divided into khalisa and istimrar as follows, viz.

	Khalisa.	Number of Villages.	Quantity of Land.			
			Biggahs.	C.	C.	
1	Ajmeer, ...	78½	563888	0	0	0
2	Kekree, ...	1	15000	0	0	0
	Istimrar.					
3	Pesangun, ...	17	148193	11	0	0
4	Bhinae, ...	80	454957	0	0	0
5	Jhooneya, ...	39	244143	0	0	0
6	Deogong Bhugera, ..	5	Unmeasured.			
7	Mussooda, ...	41	349398	0	0	0
8	Khurwah, ...	12	75490	0	0	0
9	Phooleyah, ...	68	Unmeasured.			
10	Sawur, ...	27	Unmeasured.			

The population of the district of Ajmeer is distributed as follows, according to the census taken in 1837.

District.	Pergunahs. Names.	Pergunahs. Population.	Towns and Villages marked in the map having more than 4000 inhabitants. Names.	Towns and Villages marked in the map having more than 4000 inhabitants. Population.	Number of Villages, of not more than 4000 inhabitants, in each Purgunah. Uslee Khalsee.	Daklee Khalsee.	Shamlee Khalsee.	Jaghire Villages.	Total.	Grounds on which statement or estimate of population has been made.
Ajmeer.	1 Ajmeer Proper, .	23,432	..	..	..	3	..	..	3	According to the census taken A. D. 1837, in the month of December.
	2 Pokhur, ...	9228	..	..	3	5	..	11	19	
	3 Gungwana, ...	10,866	1 Ajmeer Proper,	23,432	13½	..	..	18½	32	
	4 Hurwara, ...	2130	2 Kekree, ...	4025	3	..	..	..	3	
	5 Ramsir, ...	21,569	3 Pokhur, ...	4334	39½	8	..	17½	65	
	6 Pesangun, ...	15,740	4 Pesangun, ...	4174	10	11	..	12	33	
	7 Mussooda, ...	20,599	5 Shapoora, ...	5000	53	40	..	..	93	
	8 Rajgurh, ...	12,340	6 Sawur, ...	4100	23½	16	..	2½	42	
	9 Bhinae, ...	27,340	..	..	80	11	..	2	93	
	16 Kekree, Phooleya, Sawur, }	67,080	..	..	137	21	1	..	159	
					362½ +6				542 +6	
	Total, ...	210,324	6	45,065	368½	115	1	63½	548	

Superintendent's Office, Ajmeer, 8th April, 1838.

(Signed) J. D. MACNAGHTEN,
Superintendent of Ajmeer.

Towns. Of the towns, Ajmeer, Kekree, Shapoora, and Sawur, are walled: the "Shur-punna" of Ajmeer and of Kekree, were built by the British Government since 1818.

Borders. This district is bounded to the north-westward by Marwar; to the southward by Mewar, Harowtee, and Jaepoor; to the westward by Mewar and Marwar, and to the eastward by Kishengurh and Jaepoor.

Cantonment. Nearly south-westward of the city of Ajmeer, is the large cantonment of Nusseerabad. I shall not, however, make any remarks regarding that station, which may perhaps be considered worthy of a separate account by some one well acquainted with the immediate localities: and being removed from my individual duty, so doing might perhaps appear an intrusion to those medical residents, who are so much more capable of rendering a proper account.

Rivers. The only stream deserving the name of river, is the Kharinuddee, which skirts the district to the south-westward, dividing it from Mewar. This river is named from containing a quantity of "Khar" or carbonate of soda: when in flood, the whole water contains this salt: at other times, portions are "Khari," and the remainder not so. The water also contains a considerable proportion of muriate of soda. During the cold and hot seasons, the bed of this river has a small running stream in some places, but is in general quite dry. Water, is, however, speedily obtained by digging any where in the bed of this river. By thus digging in certain places, at remote distances, sweet water is obtained, containing only a very little muriate of soda; but in general the water is quite undrinkable and rejected in consequence of the quantity of carbonate of soda in it. This is a wide stream in the rainy season, and runs into the Bunas.

The other streams are of the nature of rain torrents: these are numerous, and during heavy rain become very impetuous, and sometimes dangerous to travellers; but soon subside again.

Near the different ridges of hills, the roads, being the lowest levels, become torrents also during heavy rain.

The Looni river rises from the Ana-sagur at Ajmeer, as a rain torrent.

There are no bodies of water that form natural lakes. Talaos are, however, numerous at almost every village, the natives being anxious to retain all the water they possibly can command. Almost every one of these talaos dries up towards the close of the cold weather. Lakes.

Three of these artificial pieces of water are, however, highly worthy of observation.

The first of these is the Ana-sagur of Ajmeer proper. This was formed by Ana Rao, grandson to Beesila-deva, by building a strong pukka bund of stone masonry, from north to south, from the "Môrie" hill to the "Sujid Silar," thus restraining the water of three considerable rain torrents, one of which only has a name, the "Bharie-nuddee." Ana-sagur.

The bund is about 600 yards in length by 100 yards in breadth, and is extremely solid and strong. Fronting to the water it is 22½ feet in height, from the foundation to the moulding; to the eastward it is much higher, and bounded by a garden called the "Dowlut bagh."

With exception of the comparatively small bund, this lake is not indebted to art; it lies between the "Nag-puhar" range, and the eastern side of the hills on which Ajmeer is built. The valley is fully three miles wide from the bund to the Poshkur pass: and is several miles in length, bounded on both sides by steep and picturesque ridges. The length of the lake is from north to south, and the breadth from east to west. In a favorable rainy season the circumference is upwards of six miles, and it then forms a large and most beautiful body of water. The deepest portion is that near the bund, varying at the greatest height, from 15 to 20 feet: and from the bund the water shoals very gradually in every direction. During the hot season, after two preceding years of insufficient rains, the Ana-sagur has been known to dry up altogether. This is computed to happen about once in fifteen years. On such occasions the malaria from the decomposing fish, insects and vegetable matters, has been very deleterious, and the effluvia very disgusting. In ordinary years the lake towards the termination of the hot winds becomes very low, averaging three feet in depth, and being one and a half mile long, by half a mile wide. The water is then green with minute floating vegetation, and larger water-plants: and also contains a large quantity of fish and insects: at this time a slight fetid effluvia is perceived. The water contains a considerable quantity of carbonate and muriate of soda; but not so much as to be quite undrinkable. In October the lake is clear and deep, and many natives then drink of it.

The dry hot winds rapidly absorb the water of the lake: and as these blow from the westward, a very pleasant diminution of temperature is felt on the bund to the eastward, producing an effect on the air very favourable to vegetation in the vicinity, and a most refreshing change to the human subject; but as this cooled current of air passes rapidly away almost due eastward, over a course of heated sand and stone, the effect is very limited and transient: and as the city lies to the north of this current no benefit is there derived, to the increase of the general salubrity.

On emerging from the pass leading from Nusseerabad to Ajmeer, it is a common observation that the air is much cooler, and this change is attributed to the influence of the Ana-sagur; but this idea appears to me much more probably to depend on the contrast between the close heated air of the pass, and the breeze generally met with on descending into the plain. It is indeed evident that no general effect can be produced on the surrounding sandy tracts of country, by so small a body of water.

The influence of the lake, however, on those who reside on the bund is very considerable, the air being more agreeable to the feelings, as well as lower in temperature.

Malaria is, no doubt extricated all round the shallow margins of the lake, from the mixture of moist earth, with decomposing animal and vegetable matters which there exist: and I conceive, that a residence to the north, south, or west of the lake would be unhealthy.

Malaria is wafted by the breeze, during the nights, towards the bund, especially in October and November; but the water is deepest at the bund, which is also considerably elevated with the buildings above the water: and those residents who keep their doors closed at night do not suffer from fever; but, I have repeatedly observed that where the reverse practice is pursued, the inhabitants become unhealthy and liable to fevers. Malaria.

The low ground in the vicinity of the bund, receiving the descending miasmata, is very unhealthy to those natives who sleep there during the rains and the early part of the cold season.

The lake contains an abundance of small eatable fish, the largest of which is the "Sowl:" all the fish keep on the increase, notwithstanding the increasing persecution of flocks of pelicans, cormorants, divers, and cranes of many kinds. Large flocks of grey geese, ducks and teal, visit the lake during the cold season. Water snakes are very abundant. Fish.

The lake has gradually much diminished in depth: and the alluvial deposits, as the water dries up, are cultivated with crops of barley and melons. The ground yields abundantly, and is the right of the "Tailies" (oilman) of Ajmeer.

A large quantity of soda is contained in the alluvial deposits, and also around the light sandy margins, where this salt effloresces abundantly on the surface during the cold season; the term "rheo mittie" is applied to soils of this nature. Soda.

The water is run off for purposes of irrigation, and to supply the dry wells by numerous small canals of masonry. The gardeners and others pay at the rate of C. Rs. 1-8-0 for watering each biggah. This tax yields the government a very small revenue. Great waste takes place in running off the water. Irrigation.

The lake, the bund, the plain and the hills, combine to form a most beautiful scene: most especially when the water is very high; yet also beautiful at any period of the rains or after, when the country is still green with vegeta- Scenery.

tion. The lake has also this further advantage, of being a fine piece of water for sailing upon.

Ghaut. A handsome and extensive ghaut, nearly adjoining the bund, has been built by Rampersaud Seth.

Suggestions. It appears to me that at a small expense, this lake might be much improved and beautified, and even prevented drying up; if the Government would redeem the ground to the north, south, and west, by paying a small price to the "Tailies," and dividing it into allotted portions, make over each in grant to wealthy individuals, on the condition of gardens being formed and kept up in good order. To such gardens dry dikes might be formed from the stone on the spot, and the intervals between filled up with the rich alluvial soil from the bed of the lake. In this earth almost every flower and fruit tree will grow with luxuriance. The supply of water would be ample; the more especially as the advance of the garden dikes into the lake, and the removal of the alluvial bed, would contract and much deepen the body of water.

A small and easily constructed floating dredging machine, would at a trifling cost, worked by three or four men, constantly deepen the lake, and increase and fertilize the surrounding gardens: the expense being paid by those receiving the supply of soil at the time.

At the same time the water should on no account be run off, except in small quantities to supply wells.

Supposing such a plan effected, owing to the extent and situation of this now neglected lake, a most enchanting scene might be produced: a real blessing would also be conferred on the city of Ajmeer, where vegetables and fruits are in general scarce, bad and dear: and where the poor are compelled to be content with their hard, dry, unpalatable, bujra, or barley bread alone.

The government might easily forego the trifling revenue, arising from selling the water for irrigation: as the only gardens thus supplied, all contain wells, which are constantly full of water by subterraneous percolation from the lake. The proprietors should therefore draw water from these wells by bullocks. A very great and useless waste of water would thus be avoided, which must inevitably take place in running off the water over the surface in a considerable stream.

The Looni has its origin from the northern end of the bund of the Ana-sagur, when in a heavy rainy season, the water overflows: and also from an artificial cut through the rock beyond. This small stream, called Sagur-mattie, flows first to the Beesila-talao, and again from thence passes to Bhowtuh and Pes-angun, where it takes a sweep northwards, and at Govindgurh is joined by the Surasvati from Poshkur, and at this "Sungum" takes the name of Looni; which does not become salt (with *muriates* of soda) till some way beyond Govindgurh. The Looni.

The second in point of magnitude is the Beesila-talao, which is entirely artificial, and was excavated upwards of a century previous to the formation of the Ana-sagur, by the emperor whose name it bears; it is situated upwards of a mile north-east of the Ana-sagur, and half a mile due east of the city of Ajmeer. The form is a regular oval, surrounded by banks and small hills formed of the earth and stones dug out. When first made, it was faced with stones and flights of steps all round; of which at present only a few traces remain. To the east is still a pukka wall and "Chudder" to allow any excess of water to escape. This talao is about 2½ miles in circumference: and must have been formed at a vast expenditure of money and labour: the bottom is said to have been perfectly level at the first construction, and the water the same depth throughout. In the centre are two small mounds forming islands. Formerly this lake received the whole water that now supplies the Ana-sagur, besides that of the large rain torrents of the adjacent hills, and also that from Taraghur, which runs through the city: at the time alluded to the Beesila-talao must have been a very large body of water; now, however, it only receives the two latter mentioned torrents, except on the rare occasions when the Ana-sagur overflows. Beesila-Talao.

The bed is much filled up by alluvial deposit, and yields

good crops of barley, when it becomes dry. After the rains, the water rapidly disappears; even after heavy rains, only a small shallow portion being retained to the eastward, during the year.

The water is much of the same quality as that of the Ana-sagur; but, owing to its so frequently drying up, and thus containing much less vegetable and animal matter, less malarious exhalation is given off during exsiccation.

When full of water the Beesila-talao is a beautiful object, and a fine view of the city is obtained from the eastward of it.

Poshkur. The third piece of water deserving mention, is the Holy Lake of Poshkur (sacred to "Brumha," the Creator; being the only lake so devoted) situated six miles west and by north of Ajmeer. The road to this lake is rather romantic; the small ghaut of the Ana-sagur is first to be passed over, affording a very pleasing view; the road then runs across the valley to the pass in the Nag-puhar range, distant three miles: this pass is a wide zigzag causeway paved with massive stones: the ascent and descent slope at an angle of about 25 degrees: thus camels lightly laden and even light carts can pass over. A fine new road, rather longer, but practicable for heavily laden carts has just been constructed by the superintendent, Mr. MacNaghten. Beyond the pass the old road runs between two ranges of hills partially wooded and green, over the heavy sandy bed of a rain torrent; the nearer the approach to Poshkur, the heavier becomes the sand.

This lake was excavated by the last of the Purihar Ranas of Mundore, and is the most sacred in India; that of Munsurwar in Thibet may alone compete with it in this respect.

Tradition records that the Sudra bildars who were employed to excavate this lake, were received into the class of brahmuns, under the title of Poshkurna or Pokhurna: and that in consequence, the "Kudharie" (or pickaxe) was amongst the articles they worshipped: and that Pokhur in Marwar was their head-quarters. It appears to be probable from what I have collected that this tradition is correct;

but, the Pokhurna brahmuns, now numerous and much respected, will not allow that it is true. Brahmuns in general are very superficially acquainted with their own origin or institutions: and considering the wound to their pride, it is but natural that the Pokhurna brahmuns should deny their origin.

The town and lake of Poshkur form a romantic scene, especially during and after the rains: the site is central to the valley, which there becoming wider, affords ample space for the numerous temples and cenotaphs, which the bigoted or devout have erected, either from pure religious motives, or as an atonement for crimes: many small palaces also adorn the margin.

Poshkur is immediately surrounded by low extensive sand hills: except to the eastward, where a swamp extends to the base of the more distant hills.

The form of the lake is irregularly elliptical: it is of considerable depth, and never dries up. A good many large alligators live in it, and are not allowed to be molested. Water-lilies, both yellow, pink, and white, abound in the shallow parts. The Puthera (or bull-rush) is plentiful and is used to make mats of.

The surrounding buildings are much interspersed with trees, which greatly enhance the beauty of the scene, contrasted with the barren sandy waste beyond and around, and forming a perfect "oasis." The connexion of ghauts and temples is only wanting on the marshy side. Every great Hindoo family endeavours to erect or possess a shrine at Poshkur; the architecture, from the different periods of construction, is very various. The most conspicuous buildings are those of Raja Maun of Jaepoor, Aheliya Baie, the Holkar queen, Jowahir Mull of Bhurtpoor, and Beejy Singh of Marwar. Jey Appa who was assassinated at Nagore, and Suntajee, who was killed during the siege of that town, are buried in a rather handsome mausoleum here.

The largest temple, a little removed from the lake, is a modern erection, the shrine dedicated to the creator Brumha, built by Gokul Paruk, the minister to Scindiah, some few years since. It cost the small sum of 130,000 Rs.; the materials were at hand, and labour on so sacred a work was to be had for almost nothing. The "Sikra" (or pinnacle) of this temple is in the form of a cross, in which circumstance there is nothing extraordinary, the cross forming a common "Sikra" or "Kulus" to sacred Hindoo structures.

The town contains two thousand houses, generally small, regular and built of stone; amongst which are three hundred shops.

Sacred Period. Every full moon is a holy time to bathe at Poshkur, and so doing obtains a remission of sins. Many other occasions also are taken advantage of as peculiarly holy periods. Two considerable fairs are held at this place: that in October is a very considerable one, the full moon of this month being a most holy time, and drawing together a great multitude of people. A great number of camels, horses, bullocks, and cows are brought for sale, and are of a superior quality. Some British troops attend to keep the peace. This fair time is the most disagreeable at which to visit Poshkur on account of various nuisances, of which the dust is neither last nor least.

Ancient Tradition. The brahmunical tradition regarding the peculiar sanctity of this spot, and its dedication to Brumha, is, that before the creation of man begun, Brumha assembled all the deities at Poshkur and performed the "Yuga:" walls or "Kanauts" were raised around the sacred spot, and sentinels placed to prevent the intrusion of evil spirits. In testimony of the fact, four isolated hills are pointed out, placed towards the cardinal points, on the summits of which hills the "Kanauts" were secured: that to the south is called "Rutnagir" (or the hill of gems) on whose top is the shrine of Sawuntri: that to the north is "Nilagir" (or the blue hill): to the east is Kutchaetar-gir: and to the west is "Sonachooru" (or the golden heap). Nanda, the bull of Mahadeva, was placed at the mouth of the valley to keep off the evil spirits of the desert, and Kaniya or Krishna guarded the north; the sacred fire was kindled; but the goddess Sawuntri, whose office it was to attend the sacred flames, as the wife of

Brumha, was no where to be found at the time, and as without a female, the rites of "Yuga" could not proceed, a young "Goozarin" was made to take her place. Sawuntri on her return was so enraged at the indignity offered to her, that she retired to the hill of gems, and disappeared in the ground, whence a fountain sprung up, which still gushes forth close to her temple, which is small, but ancient. During these rites of Brumha, Mahadeva, or, as he is called, Bhola-nath, being as usual intoxicated, omitted to put out the sacred fire, which spread and was likely to involve the world in combustion, when Brumha extinguished the fire with sand: and hence the reputed origin of the numerous "Teebas" or sandhills in the valley.

This fanciful and absurd tradition is devoutly believed by the Hindoos.

In after ages, one of the Purihar sovereigns of Mundore, in the eagerness of the chase was led to the spot, and happening to wash his hands in Sawuntri's fountain, was cured of some cutaneous disorder. In order that he might know the place again, he tore his turban to shreds and hung them on the trees. (Hence the probable origin of the custom of Hindoo pilgrims and travellers, hanging shreds of their clothes on "Chaokur" trees, met with at various spots on the roads in India; the tree in question being still very abundant about Poshkur). Here Nahur Rao, the Purihar ultimate sovereign, excavated the present lake: and the brahmuns pretend to have a grant of the surrounding land from that Rana.

Two lakes have been excavated; the old or "Boorha Poshkur" is now deserted; it lies four miles to the eastward.

The small river Sarasvati runs from Poshkur lake, and is full of "Puthera" (bull-rushes) ten or twelve feet long. Sarasvati.

The Sambhur salt lake, though not in the district of Ajmeer, is partly in the hands of our Government, under a superintendent who resides at Sambhur. Sambhur Lake.

This lake is named, according to some from the Sanskrit word "Sambhara," signifying a store: others derive the name from Sacambari-Mata, to whom there is a very ancient temple dedicated, on a hill in the middle of the lake.

Town The town of Sambhur is large, and has improved under British rule; the country around is very sandy and desolate towards Ajmeer S. W.; but is more fertile and hilly on the opposite side N. E.

The Sambhuri Sumoondr (or sea) is, after a good rainy season, about thirty miles long by ten broad, and is shallow, varying from two to fifteen feet in depth: at this season the water is not very salt.

Salt. No salt springs are known to run into, or to exist in the lake. Fresh water is found all round the margin, very near the surface. In the dry season, by digging in the bed to the depth of a few feet, a very strong brine is obtained by percolation from above into the pit, and this brine is raised and spread over a considerable surface, by which process salt is still procured, when it otherwise could not be made. It is generally believed at Sambhur that, by digging deeply in the dry bed during the hot season, fresh water can be procured, and that the stratum of salt is only superficial.

In the cold and dry season the lake rapidly dries up: and only a portion of a few miles in extent contains water; which is white on the surface with crystallized salt, as is also the dry bed; thus an immense snow-white expanse, waving with "mirage," produced by heated currents of air, presents a remarkable spectacle to the eye.

At this time, strong salt brine is found by digging only a few inches in the dry bed: the solution is coloured red apparently by oxide of iron: the brine is run off into large "Kearies" (spaces fenced in) in the bed of the lake: and when sufficient has accumulated, it is left to evaporate and deposit crystals: at length the brine remains only about one foot in depth, and the chloride of sodium is copiously spread over the bottom in a mass of crystals.

The salt is now removed, and raised up into enormous heaps around the margins of the lake, and being well beaten down, does not perceptibly diminish during the heaviest rain.

After the cubicular crystals of common salt have been precipitated, a large quantity of prismatic crystals of sulphate of soda are formed below, which might be applied to many useful purposes, such as cooling wine, or by decomposition the production of pure soda. Sulphate of Soda.

The Sambhur lake has yielded salt during a long series of ages, in undiminished quantities.

The surrounding country contains an abundance of soda; but very little salt: yet as the salt in the lake itself seems superficial, it can only remain to suppose that the supply of salt is washed in during the rains: however, all the entering streams have been examined, and none were found to be saline.

Geological researches, especially by boring, around and in the bed of this lake, would prove very interesting: as, whence the vast, inexhaustible supply of salt is produced, is a very just subject of curiosity.

The absence of any apparent source has given rise to the *native* belief, that the "nimmuk" is formed in the soil or water, from the "khar" (carbonate of soda): however, this cannot be the case, as no other muriates exist, that would be decomposed by the soda, to form the supply of salt in any thing like sufficient quantities: the only one being muriate of lime in very minute portion.

The wells in the Ajmeer district, though sufficiently abundant for ordinary purposes, are, on the whole, far too few. Wells.

Many tracts of country, which would yield an excellent rubbee crop by irrigation, are allowed to lie fallow during that season, owing to the want of wells; I allude especially to the country about Kekree, where the soil is very good, yet by far the greatest part of the crop is "Khureef" only.

There is certainly not a more beneficent object open to the Government, nor one which would be more gratefully appreciated by the natives, than that of digging numerous wells in this district, and defraying the expense by a remission of the revenue: and the Government would certainly gain in the end by increase of produce and population.

The wells are of various depths: in the sandy low moist grounds (called "Sirs") much impregnated with saline matters, the water is near the surface, and in general is "Khari" and bad: those dug through the rock are much deeper and the water is purer.

A great many of the more shallow wells become dry during the hot season: and in very dry seasons also a number of those dug through the superior strata of rocks. The soil of the district is eminently adapted for percolation down to the first strata of rocks: and, it would appear, that the water is only retained in the sandy wells, and also in those in the superficial rocks, by the firm resistance of the rocky sub-strata; hence, when the moisture of the soil and approximate schistose rocks is exhausted, a very general scarcity of water is the result, causing the greatest distress.

Therefore, in digging wells, there is one fact worthy of the greatest attention; this is, that abundance of pure water is always to be obtained below the solid white quartzoze rock, underlying the hornblende schist, which in this district is so frequently met with. The natives, informed on this subject, state that, after digging through the sand, a light yellow loam is found, then concrete carbonate of lime or marl ("Moorur" and "Dhobi mittie"), then hornblende schist, which latter has to be passed through a considerable depth, of from 60 to 70 feet, when white solid quartz is generally found: and on this occurring, it is common to congratulate the owner of the well, saying, "Now blow up the white rock, and you have water for ten biggahs of land." The quartz is solid, about ten feet in thickness, and is very difficult to get through; but, when once removed *water rises in abundance, never fails and is of good quality.* Instead, therefore, of resting satisfied at obtaining a precarious supply of "Khari" water above; it would be better to dig on till the quartz is reached: this should be done at least in two wells in every village, and a never failing supply of pure water would be obtained.

By far the greater number of the wells in the Ajmeer district are at present "Khari;" which term has no relation to common salt, but is alone applied to signify the fossil alkali or carbonate of soda: on the contrary, the water of springs containing common salt is called, "Nimkin panee" or "Loonki."

The "Khari" water is not objectionable for crops of wheat or barley: indeed, the latter grain is said to thrive better when so irrigated. Many fruit trees and some flowers are killed by the use of Khari water; therefore, a sweet water well is a great desideratum in gardens. Many villages contain one or two wells of what is called sweet water; but, which, in fact, is only less "Khari" than that of the other wells. The natives will not drink "Khari" water, if they can possibly avoid doing so, as it purges them, giving pain in the intestines, and causing indigestion; especially if habitually used. This is a curious fact; compared with the knowledge, that large quantities of carbonate of soda, are habitually and with impunity used as an antacid remedy by many dyspeptic subjects during a series of years; which may perhaps be accounted for by the general absence of acid, in the stomachs of the natives, leaving the alkali free to exert a deleterious effect; or, more probably to the presence of lime in the same water.

Curious Fact.

The "Khari" water is in appearance clear, is destitute of odour, and has a strong simply alkaline, and not at all saltish taste. The addition of a minute portion of acid, causes a perceptible disengagement of carbonic acid gas, so abundant is the carbonate of soda: nitrate of silver throws down a faint white cloud (chloride of silver) indicating the presence of a minute portion of common salt: the taste, however, is not in the least saline, and the natives assert that there is no salt in "Khari panee:" oxalic acid throws down a faint precipitate, proving the presence of a very little lime. This water is soft and good for washing; but, the soap soon separates and comes to the surface, owing to the little lime in solution.

Scarcity of Wells. Some villages contain no wells, owing to their poverty: in one, near Ajmeer, there has been little or no rubbee crop for ten years past, and only a Khurreef crop in a good rainy season: facts, such as this, not uncommon, are very disheartening to the poor ryots.

Best Water. The most coveted water at the city of Ajmeer, is that of the "Koomar bowlie," the "Lakha bowlie" the "Khatun bowlie" and the "Doodiya Kooa," in or near the city, and the "Tailee ka Kooa" on the eastern side of the Ana-sagar. The natives declare these waters are very light and sweet; but the fact, by analysis, is, that they all contain a small portion of common salt perceptible to the taste on reflection, and which renders the water more agreeable to the palate than the perfectly pure fluid would be. On the addition of nitrate of silver, the chloride of that metal is faintly precipitated in each specimen of water.

Morasses. Bogs. There are no real morasses in this district; but there are many low-lying sandy portions of land, in which water is very near the surface, especially after the rains. The saline particles of the surrounding country are washed into these grounds by the heavy rains, and by their affinity for moisture, give the surface, even in the dry season, a damp appearance. Hardly any vegetation but dhoop grass is apparent in such places, which are generally denominated "Sir," from their moisture; but I have not heard that they are considered as causes of unhealthiness at any time.

Saline Efflorescence. In the cold and hot weather, the surfaces of these places, are, in many parts, white with saline efflorescence, chiefly carbonate of soda with aluminous earth. The impure soda is called "Reeah," and earth so impregnated "Reeoh mittie," found almost every where in Upper India; but very common at Ajmeer: where, in some parts of the district it may be collected in quantities by the hand even. The taste is mildly alkaline and not salt. The Dhobis collect it in quantities, and either use it plain in washing, or make it into soap.

Remarkable Fact. It is remarkable, in a country so much abounding in felspar and mica, perpetually undergoing natural decomposition, that so very small a proportion of the salts of potash should be found in these saline grounds.

Potash only appears to be found combined with nitric acid in the vicinity of villages, in those places where azotized substances (such as bones and other animal matters) have accumulated during a series of years: and from the sweepings of such places saltpetre is obtained: the potash in this instance being supplied from the felspar or mica of the soil. Potash.

After the "Reeah" or effloresced soda has been removed from these saline grounds, the "Kharie nimmuk" is obtained by lixiviating the under sweepings. Notwithstanding the goodness and cheapness of the Sambhur salt, the "Kharie nimmuk" is frequently made in this district and used by the poorer villagers by way of economizing: and is much given to cattle. Kharie nimmuck

An inferior caste, called "Kharol" from the employment, manufacture this salt: in other parts of India "Noniya" is a common name applied to this caste. Kharol Caste.

The sweepings are collected in a considerable mass, by the side of a shallow well dug in the sand for the purpose: an earthen gurra, attached by a rope to a balanced pole, is used to raise the water: about 50 maunds of sweepings are accumulated, and then 10 or 12 gurras of water are poured on the heap, and this process frequently repeated: the heap sloaps behind to a narrow channel, leading to a shallow reservoir of stone and mortar, into which, the water gradually percolating from the heap, runs and evaporates. First, a pellicle, more or less consistent, forms on the surface, consisting of impure soda mixed with salt; this is removed by the hand skimming it off, and is sold as "Khar" or alkali, and is used by "Chumars" to dress leather with, and also given as medicine to sheep and other animals: the crystals of chloride of sodium are deposited below; they are dirty reddish coloured, and impure, containing muriate of lime, rendering the taste austere and bitter; and from this cause the "Kharie or Bhukea nimmuk" is partially deliquescent during the rains, and will not do to preserve meat. Very Process.

considerable quantities are manufactured. Fifty maunds of sweepings may yield twenty seers of salt.

It is curious, that the sweepings in question, have a strongly alkaline taste, and a very faint salt one.

On this account the "Kharols" suppose that the salt is formed from the soda during the process.

The product of chloride of sodium is certainly much greater than the soil of the "Sirs" seems to contain: and the product in no degree diminishes. The surrounding soil contains free soda much more abundantly than common salt.

Source of the Salt.

However, there can remain no doubt that the salt is âb initio, derived from the soil, though its existence is not very evident; there being no apparent or even probable source for the supply of muriatic acid or chlorine to form the combination.

Mountains.

The only elevations, worthy of the name of mountains, in the Ajmeer district, are Taraghur; immediately overlooking the city, and within the semi-oval formed by two spurs of which Ajmeer is situated; the Mudar range (so named from possessing a "Durgah" sacred to a Mahommedan saint) running in a line north and south, and rising a mile and a half east of the town walls, and only a little inferior in elevation to Taraghur; and the range that separates the Ajmeer district from the Mairwarra, (a part of the Aravulli) may be considered as mountainous.

Hills.

The other numerous elevations are more or less scattered in very irregular ranges, of no great length, and separated by plains: and they rather deserve the name of considerable hills, than mountains. The highest of these are the Bhinae range, and the Nag-puhar range near Ajmeer itself.

The hills are most numerous and approximate more closely near the city, than elsewhere in the district.

Geological Character.

The general character of the rocks composing the mountains and hills, is primitive: and their individual nature is schistose in the greatest proportion; the strata lying obliquely, dipping from east to west: the fracture is often perpendicular to the surface; they abound in seams, containing "Moorur" (carbonate of lime) or yellow ochry earth: in many places they are exceedingly disintegrated, composed of debris of quartz, mica, felspar, schorl, and yellow ochry soil.

It is evident that hills of this character must absorb and retain a vast quantity of water in the innumerable crevices, through which the water very slowly percolates; so much so is this the case, that the rain absorbed only reaches the general level of the country in April or May; at which time, after a favorable season, the Lall-Diggee is usually overflown, yielding a timely supply. Retentive of Water.

This quantity of water in the hills, after favorable rains, must in some degree modify the subsequent temperature.

There are other hills of a less absorbent character: such as the lower part of the Sat-poora range, composed of rolled masses of quartz with hornblende and schorl; and granite of different kinds, especially near to Shapoora, and Suk-rani.

Taraghur is a table mountain, elevated between 1,000 and 1,100 feet above the plain below. This is, I think, a near approximation to the absolute height; though, I am aware, that the height has been considered by some not to exceed 800 feet. Considering my calculation as correct, the elevation of Taraghur above the sea is upwards of 3,000 feet, the plain of Ajmeer being 2,000 feet above the sea level. Taraghur.

The surface is completely walled around, and is irregular, much longer than broad, and having a long very narrow salient angle to the south. The circumference of the walls is two miles. The fort is approached by inclined planes of great length, at a considerable angle, roughly paved and parapetted; by which, when formerly in repair, guns and horses could be taken up. This ascent is well covered by the fort itself, and also by outworks and the hill to the west. The fort contains one large and one smaller tank, and commands another outside. During the time when the fort was held as a military post, the tank water was preserved for emergencies: and all the usual supply for the garrison, was brought by "Bhesties" from below, up the long and toilsome ascent.

The ancient name of Taraghur was Gurh-beetli: the fort

at first was of much smaller extent, when erected by the Purihar Rajpoots; these most ancient portions are still seen, and are formed of very massive square stones, so large that popular belief assigns their position to the labour of the "deities:" several of the Purihar watch-towers still remain on the spurs of Taraghur; they are square and unsightly; but are extremely massive.

Extensive Remains. When Aja-Pal, the Chohan, took possession, he completed, by the aid of his race, not only the fortifications of Beetli-gurh; but also of the adjacent hills, along the ridges of which massive walls extend for miles. Where the hill was not naturally sufficiently steep, it has been scarped. Altogether the labour bestowed has been on a very grand scale.

Considered Impregnable. When the fort was taken by Allah-ood-deen, the gates and battlements were repaired: and it was long considered impregnable. The Chohan Rajpoots, however, of Rajghur, on one occasion assembled, and escaladed the place by surprise, though they did not keep possession long.

Dismantled. Taraghur was finally dismantled by order of Lord W. Bentinck. It is still, however, a strong place and capable of repair.

Durgah. A durgah of white marble on the top is sacred to Moyen-ud-deen, dependent on the greater durgah below sacred to the same saint. The view from the durgah is very extensive and in the rainy season is beautiful.

Khadims. About 250 Khadims with their families reside on Taraghur, and are supported by the proceeds of several small jaghires granted by the first Subahdur, Meera Saheb, and by the emperors Ackber Shah, Jehangire, and Mahomed Shah; and also by Hindoo princes. There are about sixty houses inhabited on Taraghur. The Khadims look generally clean and respectable: they are quite idle: their houses and families are in a wretched condition.

The great durgah is situated at the foot of Taraghur, in the town of Ajmeer, and is formed of a neat assemblage of plain white marble buildings, and paved courts. There is nothing imposing in the appearance. On this far celebrated shrine, by far the greater number of Khadims are dependent: and the chief jaghires and donations are attached. The bones of the saint Kwaja Moyen-ud-deen are contained in a small mausoleum.

The saint is equally a favorite with Hindoos and Mahommedans, and can be equally propitiated by both. The worship seems a "meleè" of Hindoo and Islamite rites. A great annual fair is held in October in the saint's honor, and a smaller one later in the season. Some attempt at shew is kept up; and people flock to the fair from all quarters. Miracles are openly pretended: the most absurd impositions are practised, especially in the great tent erected for the occasion, in which a little rolling about, and foaming at the mouth, pass for the inspiration of the saint's spirit. Offerings are also tied in turbans or "kummerbunds," and suspended to the trees, by parties chiefly Hindoos, the other ends of the cloths being retained by the votaries who sleep under the trees; and it is a general belief that on whatsoever account the offering is made, the wish will be granted. In many instances these wishes are very trifling, and the Khadims easily manage to ascertain the object desired, from some of the parties, and then contrive to slip unseen the article wished for into the cloth suspended to the tree, during the sleep of the party, who on awaking, in foolish astonishment soon spreads abroad the new miracle. All the numerous offerings of other parties are removed, *their* wishes not being obtained on account of their *sins!*

Kwaja Moyen-ud-deen.

Fair.

Kwaja Moyen-ud-deen was a native of Sinjur; he is stated to have become a faqueer, and leaving his home came first to Delhi, and from thence to Ajmeer; where he took up his abode under some trees, where the present site of the durgah now is. At that time the hills and valley of the Ajmeer lake were covered with jungle: at one place (where the Sêth's burying-ground now is) there was an ancient shrine sacred to Mahadeva, the "lingum" of which was hidden by the leaves and rubbish. To this wood the Kwaja had retired to contemplate during forty days; and every day hung up his small "mussuq" of water on a branch of a tree overhanging the "lingum:" the water constantly dropped on this: at length Mahadeva became highly pleased, both at the sanctity and unexpected libation of the saint, and spoke out of the stone commending his virtue. From this tradition (related by one of the most learned Khadims) the Hindoos equally venerate the Kwaja with the Mahommedans.

Vast Iron Cauldrons.

Large iron deghs or pans are erected near the durgahs: and these used formerly to be often filled by devotees, with savoury viands; now, however, such an occurrence is rare. The contents of the largest would feed some thousand mouths.

Pilgrimages.

The pilgrimages, on foot, to this saint, made by the celebrated Ackber Shah, shew to what a great length superstition will on particular points lead the wisest.

Burra Peer.

On a principal spur of Taraghur is erected another more modern durgah, within a half-moon bastion, over the remains of a "Bura Peer," a faqueer who came from Bagdad, bringing (as is usual) two bricks along with him as relics; placing these under a tree he lived there with great sanctity, and at length dying during the Maharatta rule, both Hindoos and Mahommedans combined to erect the durgah; to which a small jaghire is attached. The bastion is often lighted up in the evenings: and owing to its elevation, presents a curious and pleasing spectacle.

Taraghur has been spoken of by some in authority as likely to be beneficial as a sanatarium for the sick officers and others from the cantonments of Nusseerabad.

Taraghur unfit for a Sanatarium.

My own opinion is; that as a residence it would be extremely agreeable, were a proper building erected. The elevation is not, however, sufficient to produce a great change of temperature. The surface is unequal and extensive and retains much moisture: and has abundant vegetation, giving rise to miasmatic exhalations at the usual seasons. The long, steep, circuitous ascent would almost preclude medical attendance.

Again; the temperature on Taraghur varies extremely.

Those who live there, state it as a very agreeable residence during the hot winds and rains, the former being hardly perceptible, and the nights always cool; but the sudden great variations of temperature, from great heat to moist cold, render the place far from a healthy abode.

Water is scarce and bad. The cholera very seldom visits Taraghur, even when severe in Ajmeer. Fevers are wild and not very frequent, at the usual season. The inhabitants die young: complaints of the chest are common, both asthmatic and phthisical: probably owing to the laborious steep ascent, and over-heating thus occasioned, and the common sudden variations of temperature. Guineaworm is very common.

Notwithstanding the considerable elevation and the occasional severity of thunder storms, the electric fluid has not been known to do any damage.

The hills about Ajmeer and in the district are very bare and destitute of trees. Formerly the forest and brushwood formed extensive tracts. During the 57 years' sway of the Maharattas, the wood was chiefly cut down: and this depredation forms a very general cause of complaint against that people. Trees. Scarce.

The hills would soon resume their clothing of trees, if sufficient protection were afforded to the young plants; as is especially evident on inspecting the debris of the Ajmeer lead mine, which is becoming covered with neem trees. The growth of wood on the now bare hills, would in time be highly beneficial to the health of the inhabitants, by diminishing the temperature, by radiation of heat in the night, and interception of the sun's rays during the day; at present the excessive heat often prevalent being a principal cause of disease to those much exposed.

In the month of October, when the temperature of the night differs much from that of the day, the air contained in the concavities of the hills, becomes much cooled during the nights, when wind is not prevalent; and at sun-rise, when a breeze generally rises, these cool portions mingling with warmer currents of air, give rise to very disagreeable Currents of Air.

sensations on being met with, and are thought to be very unwholesome. In Sicily similar draughts of air from the "fuimari" are much dreaded.

Euphorbia. Thuar (euphorbia) is very abundant on many of the hills and plains below: and its presence seems dependent on the quantity of carbonate of lime (mur rur) in the soil.

Climate. In comparison with other parts of India where I have resided, either to the southward, eastward, or northward, the climate of Ajmeer town and district is exceedingly salubrious. The general character is that of great dryness. The hot wind commences about the end of March or beginning of April, and blows strongly and steadily day and night till the early part or middle of June. During all this time the temperature is very high; but, to those who can employ the cooling aid of tatties, this season is very agreeable: and even by the community who are at all sheltered a great exemption from disease is experienced: to this rule, there are two exceptions; the one is variola, which generally appears in March, and often becomes dreadfully fatal, at this season; the other embraces those cases arising from direct exposure of individuals to the sun's powerful rays, a very frequent cause of disease and death.

The city of Ajmeer is oppressively hot at this season, being situated directly under and to the west of Taraghur and the adjacent hills: thus greatly exposed to reflected heat: and the breeze, when light, being often totally intercepted. The wind, however, generally blows with such violence as to surmount every obstacle: and the westerly rays of the sun are intercepted at an early period of the afternoon by the hills alluded to.

The houses of the officers, civil and military, are situated at a distance from the town, and are fairly exposed to the influence of the climate. A very small degree of sickness has occurred at any time in those residences. The magazine, connected with the town, in which Europeans also dwell, has been equally exempt.

My own house was on the bund of the Ana-sagur, and the air there and in the immediate vicinity was moister, and the temperature lower: and, as I have remarked when speaking of the Ana-sagur, if a resident acts with the necessary caution of avoiding night exposure, the situation will be found exceedingly healthy and agreeable.

From the causes before explained, the influence of the Ana-sagur on the climate, is circumscribed to the bund, and directly to the leeward of it, and in no way has any advantageous effect on the town or more distant houses.

Any mists that arise from the lakes at Ajmeer during the nights in the cold season, are prevented affecting the town by the intervening range of hills, and are soon dispersed by a light breeze.

The heat during the hot winds, unmodified by a tattie, becomes very great even in the house. During three years' observations the highest temperature remarked by me, occurred in the night in May, 1838, when a strong hot wind was blowing, and the differential thermometer in the morning marked 110 degrees.

By tatties well watered, the temperature can generally be insured from 78 to 82 degrees, and is very bearable.

On the whole the climate is much less mutable than I have elsewhere observed.

The very little variation of the barometer rendered it useless to register observations: $\frac{1}{10}$ of an inch being the average variation, even during the rains. Barometer

In December, January, and February, in still clear nights, the thermometer often sinks below the freezing point: hoar frost, and ice in thin pellicles, being abundantly formed: at this period from 65° to 72° is the range of the mid-day temperature. From the early part of November to the end of February, the climate of Ajmeer is most delightful, and invigorating in a high degree: and is generally favorable to invalids, except in rheumatic or pulmonic cases. Children and others at this season present florid complexions. Exercise can be taken at almost any period of the day. Contrasted with what is experienced in many other parts of India, this season is, at Ajmeer, exceedingly pleasant, and the climate admirable. Temperature

Rainy Season. The rains commence about the middle of June, and terminate in the middle of September or early in October. The rains are much lighter and less continuous at Ajmeer, than they are to the east and south: and about every third year fall very partially, giving rise often to great distress, from an insufficient supply. The commencing showers are very heavy and soon over. The after rains are at intervals and much lighter. Three days' constant showers are very uncommon: and a day seldom occurs without a dry interval. During the longer intervals a strong westerly breeze generally blows; most refreshing to the senses, and often pleasanter from the scent of the flowering vegetation, especially the wild indigo, over which it blows. The close saturated atmosphere is not often experienced, though occasionally very close days and nights happen. Thermometer averages 84°: whenever the mercury rises to 88° or 90° rain speedily will fall.

At this season, a light vegetation springs up every where and the appearance of the country becomes very beautiful.

Deluging Rains. Twice, upon record, very deluging rains have fallen in the Ajmeer district: the one is recorded by Sir T. Roe, in the time of Jehangire: the other happened in 1831.

Diseases incidental to this season are very mild at Ajmeer: fevers are at first continued or remittent, and become more periodical as the season advances. On the whole, this, the unhealthiest season is more salubrious at Ajmeer, than the generality of the healthiest seasons of most stations to the south and east.

Meteorological Remarks. A protracted account of thermometrical observations, or other meteorological remarks, taken on the bund where my house was, would be useless, owing to the influence of the vicinity of so large a body of water on the instruments employed; I have therefore given only the average of the temperature of the station.

The houses on the bund have a temperature three degrees lower than those on the plains.

Great dryness is the general characteristic of the climate during the hot winds, and cold seasons: and comparatively in the rains also. The atmosphere during all the seasons is much agitated by strong breezes, rendering the hot weather bearable, the rains often very pleasant, and the cold season delightfully bracing.

The least accession of moisture produces a vegetation of poa and other grasses; but the verdure is never rank.

According to my observation, a stagnation of the electrical currents rarely takes place at Ajmeer; but, when this state becomes evident by the presence of a still close atmosphere and heavily surcharged clouds; it is at such times that cholera becomes epidemic: and as soon as the universal interchange of the electric currents recurs, the epidemic abates or altogether subsides. Electrical Stagnation.

Even the slightest film of vapour has the greatest effect on the temperature here, as every where else: diminishing the heat during the day, especially in the hotter season; but, at all times more than counterbalancing this effect by interruption of radiation during the night: causing in the cold months a difference of 20° of heat, compared with those days and nights when the sky is clear. The heat is especially oppressive at these times, owing to the common absence of wind. If the cholera *ever* happens to appear in the *cold* season it is at such periods that it breaks out. Radiation.

Any irregularity in the by-gone routine of the seasons, seems to have a marked power over the subsequent weather and a considerable time elapses ere the regularity is restored. Thus, if the hot winds commence early in April and blow steadily, with only one or two heavy squalls in May, the rains may be confidently expected about the 10th or 15th of June, and will set in heavily and continue at intervals till early in October: at which time there will be an abundant supply of water all over the country, and a very cold season will follow till the middle of December, about which time if one or two heavy showers (called the Mahawut) fall, and then the clouds clear up, the cold season will be diminished greatly in temperature and prolonged in duration, the crops will be splendid, and again a regular hot wind will succeed. Routine of Seasons.

On the other hand, if a considerable period of cloudy weather occurs in December, with light partial showers, the cold season will be much cut short, and become less healthy; the clouds will at length clear up, and after an interval of fifteen or twenty days again appear and light showers fall: the season will be altogether hotter, and the crops will be inferior. In March, April, and May, clouds will continue to gather, and in May generally heavy rain will fall: the hot wind will not blow freely: the season will be oppressive comparatively: the rains will not set in till the end of June, or early in July, will be light, and end about the middle of September: the following cold season will probably again be of shorter duration than usual, and hotter.

This weather may be expected every third or fourth year.

Severe Frosts. In a fine cold season, the frosts are often very severe, and tend to prevent the rapid growth of young trees in the hills.

Soils. The soil of the district may be described as being greatly conducive to the health of the inhabitants; from the absorbent quality, the absence of rank vegetation, the speedy drainage by numerous small rapid nullahs, combining to prevent the formation of the supposed causes of febrile miasmata in any great degree.

All the water that falls very speedily reaches the general level of the more superficial springs, about 20 or 30 feet from the surface: the percolation being rapid, the surface dries very soon: and in very few places does water lodge, combined with decomposing vegetable and animal matters, immediately below a deceiving dry sandy surface; such a natural arrangement as gives rise to the extrication of the most deadly miasmata in some parts of Sicily, in the isle of Ascension, and other places: on the contrary the decomposing remains are washed away and scattered with great rapidity by the rain torrents.

Rapid Percolation.

By far the greater portion of the soil of the Ajmeer district is sandy: this sand consists chiefly of disintegrated mica schist and felspar: pure silicious sand is much less common. The hills, as before mentioned, are generally schistose, and absorb much water which percolates slowly through them: externally their inclination is steep, and drainage complete: around the bases of these hills, large tracts exist of sand and gravel, of broken-down schist with masses of schist, quartz, felspar, schorl and other rocks appearing above the surface: these tracts abound in carbonate of lime, in places where the euphorbiæ are most common: barren as they appear in the dry season, both hills and adjacent tracts become covered with a delicate verdure of grasses and other small plants.

No superficial portion of the soil is absolutely clayey; but, strong bright yellow loam, containing soda, is dug out under Taraghur and in many places in the district: cretaceous and aluminous marls (the one exceeding in chalk, the other in alumina), are dug out very abundantly in many places a few feet below the surface.

Calcareous gravel or "kunkul" is plentiful in places where water flows during the rains.

No portion of the soil of this district can be considered alluvial: excepting the beds of artificial talaos, where generally a rich productive dark-coloured loam, mixed with vegetable matter, occurs.

Of the cultivated soil, these beds of talaos contain the best found in the district; but form a very small proportion.

The general run of the cultivated soil is called "bhura mittie," from its light yellow colour. This is a natural mixture of ⅓ stiff yellow loam, with ⅔ of sand of mica schist and felspar; and forms a very light soil; but yields good crops by the aid of manure, especially khurreef crops.

As this "bhura mittie" contains sand of mica schist and felspar, it is evident that in the course of time the land must improve by decomposition of the particles.

The "bhura mittie" forms only a small portion of the surface of the country.

In some places the soil is marly; and is called "dholie mittie" (or white earth): and these portions are cultivated and yield good crops: the same term is applied to that soil where uncombined carbonate of lime (moorur) abounds;

only a very small portion of which admits of being at all cultivated.

The remaining land is designated as "baloo-ret" (gravelly sand), and by the aid of much manure sometimes produces good khurreef crops of bujra. This "baloo-ret" is micaceous and felspathic.

In the beds of rivers, even the pure silicious sand, by the aid of water and plenty of manure produces a crop of barley in the cold season.

Artificial soil exists near most villages and towns, and in considerable quantity near Ajmeer.

Many "sirs" or moist saline grounds are scattered over the district.

Soil in relation to health.

The period of the year, in relation to the soil, that is most unhealthy, is here, (as elsewhere) when the rains become partial or cease: the temperature being about 80° in the day. This period generally extends at Ajmeer from the end of September to the middle of November.

The portion of land that is cultivated compared to that which lies fallow, or, has never been cultivated, is so very small, that any deleterious effect on the inhabitants of the district cannot be attributed to this cause.

Around a few of the larger towns a very considerable space is cultivated; but, in general, on surveying the country from any height, the cultivated land around the villages appears very insignificant, compared with the vast plains or low hills.

In other parts of India, the stubble left in the fields, the fallen leaves of a crop, or other remains, long continue moist, and often became rotten, over very large spaces of land; but in the Ajmeer district, from the dryness of the air and soil, the remains of the crops almost immediately become dry, and continue so until the ground is again ploughed up.

From the universal use of manure, and from the practice of irrigation, especially around the larger towns where there is much cultivation, it might perhaps seem evident that a noxious effect must be produced on the inhabitants; but, from repeated and careful inquiries it does not appear that such is the case.

That no ill effect is experienced, may, I think, be properly attributed to the facts; that the rubbee cultivation does not commence till the end of October, when the season generally becomes very healthy; that only the quantity of manure, absolutely required by the crop, is used; that each crop is only watered twice or thrice during the season, and no superfluity being expended the surface soon dries up; and that the temperature of the air does not favour the extrication of miasmata during the cold season, in this district.

Of the agricultural operations, there appear none that are peculiarly, or in any degree, unhealthy to those employed.

A small quantity of indigo is made, and the steeped plant undergoes a noisome putrefaction; but, those employed in the manufacture, though wet constantly, do not suffer from their occupation.

Agriculture.

The soil of the district being light and poor, the rainy season being also lighter than elsewhere, the agriculturists are compelled to compensate the deficiencies of nature by art. Their agricultural instruments are more numerous, and although still simple, are better adapted for effect, than is the case in more fertile regions.

The plough, the rake, the hoe, and the drilling machine (a hollow bamboo and funnel) are in common use: the pitchforks made of wood, bound with thongs, are neat and convenient. The general method of drawing water from the wells is effective and cheap: the skin of water, by a common simple contrivance of an inverted syphon (called "scor") connected to the drag-rope by a thong, emptying itself at the right moment; thus requiring the attention of only one man who drives the bullocks. Sometimes two pairs of bullocks are used alternately, the well rope being connected to the yokes by a toggle; this method is very expeditious. The carts are strong, and have the centre of gravity raised, to facilitate the passage over the stony roads: and the wheels are built with removable wooden tyres, with great economy of material. The cattle for ploughs and carts are superior. Every economical contrivance is resorted to, and is manifest in the method of stacking grain, grass, straw or bhoosa.

Manure. Excepting only in the dry beds of talaos, manure is everywhere resorted to: every kind is collected in heaps, outside the walls of the villages. This manure is used to the superior kinds of khurreef crops, and to all the rubbee crops: and as the quantity of ground cultivated depends very much on the supply of manure, this is very carefully husbanded.

Gardens. In the garden grounds, and in some of the fields near large towns, by the use of large quantities of manure, a constant succession of crops is obtained during the year: and generally when manure can be used freely, at least one good crop can be reaped during the year from any land; but everywhere else where there is a deficient supply, the land cultivated two years in succession, must be allowed to lie fallow for one year or more.

Scarcity of Manure. Could sufficient manure be commanded, as one crop only occupies the ground a few months, even the poorest soil would yield an annual crop. The want of this, however, together with the great deficiency of wells, (as stated under that head) combine to keep the quantity of land in cultivation at a low standard.

The land for khurreef crops is ploughed generally in June; but, if a heavy shower falls in April or May, immediate advantage is then taken to plough, and sow bujra or juar, which rapidly springs up, and though afterwards somewhat burnt up by the heat of these months, they survive till the regular rains in June, when they sprout forth vigorously and yield an early and abundant crop.

The cultivators are seen at the beginning of the rains taking advantage of every shower to prepare even the most inhospitable-looking ground for the seed. From the very great lightness of the soil the ploughing is easily and carelessly performed.

Rain Crops. The rain crops are chiefly bujra and juar: these being the staple grains of the country; these are generally sown without any manure, and frequently in almost pure sand: yet, a very plentiful crop sometimes results: I have many times counted from 15 to 20 stems of bujra from one root. The cultivators sow these grains very thinly by broad casts, and after the plant has attained a certain height, plough up again between the stalks.

Moth (a legume) is also extensively cultivated at this season, sown along with bujra: its produce is very variable, sometimes remaining diminutive, but in a copious rainy season spreading extensively over the ground, and yielding a large return. This moth is the staple legume of the country, and is especially used to feed horses. The flour of bujra and juar, and the "dâl" of moth, are the common diet of the poorer inhabitants: and from habit they prefer this food, so much despised by the natives of the more fertile regions of India.

The other rain crops are mukka, moong, tobacco, lobiya, til, and kupas (cotton): all of these require a quantity of manure. The mukka yields a heavy crop, and the grain is ground into flour and much used.

The rubbee cultivation commences at the end of October. Winter Crops.
The fields are well manured, spread well abroad, the dry ground is then watered, and when sufficiently dry is ploughed up, the grain is then drilled in, in rows, very thinly sown: the field is then carefully raked with large wooden rakes, and divided into small regular divisions (or kearies), having a water-course between every two lines. In the best land wheat is sown, in that less good barley is cultivated, and vastly exceeds in quantity the wheat.

In some lower darker portions of land, chenna is cultivated without irrigation.

In the best garden ground, with plenty of manure, sugar-cane is cultivated, and requires much water.

The production of all the grains, except bujra, juar and moth, requires considerable labour, on the part of the ryot; and all the products are very inferior compared with those of more fertile soils, the bujra alone excepted.

A very little rice is sown sometimes by the malees: the quantity is hardly worthy of mention.

The wheat is of an inferior quality, of a small dark-coloured grain (kutea and pisea,) yielding more gluten than is generally proportionate to the farina, and also from the thickness of the husk, a great quantity of bran. The same seed seems to have been sown in succession, time out of mind.

The barley is also inferior, small in grain and abounding in husk.

The chenna is of similar quality.

Change of Seed required.

One grain of the fine white "julaleea," dukhani wheat, outweighs more than two grains of the Ajmeer wheat, and is also a thin skinned grain, containing proper relative proportions of gluten and farina. This seed might be easily obtained from Hoshungabad, and tried at Ajmeer on an extensive scale.

As the "mukka" (or Indian corn) thrives well, and is extensively cultivated, the superior American sorts should be introduced.

The sugar-cane being only cultivated in garden ground by malees, the Otaheiti variety ought to be tried.

Suggestions regarding Manure.

As manure is so very valuable an object in this district, the attention of improvers is naturally directed to this object.

The common run of ground is the "bhura mittie" (brown yellow soil), light and sandy, with a little yellow loam; but in many places below the surface the "pandol mittie" (or cretaceous marl), is very abundant, and in other parts a strong yellow loam is plentiful, a few feet below the surface.

From such ingredients, with vegetable and animal remains, a most plentiful supply of manure might be prepared.

The inhabitants of villages should unite to form large central mounds of these materials, during the periods when cultivation is not going on. A thick layer of vegetable matter, (old straw, stalks or leaves of any kind,) should first be spread out, three feet in thickness; over this, one foot of the marl should be laid, and over that two feet of vegetable matters, old bones, and all kinds of dung: and, if possible, over this two feet of the strong yellow loam; thus, the strata should be alternated, until in time a very large heap would be produced. This heap should be allowed to remain one year exposed to the weather, so as to allow the vegetable and animal matters to decompose, and the mass to consolidate.

The whole village would then be supplied from this heap for a long period: in removing this manure with the spade or hoe, the materials should be equally incorporated.

A heap should be newly constructed in time to succeed the one being expended at the proper period.

From the liberal use of this manure, the land would be permanently and greatly improved.

As the necessity for irrigation in this district is universal, the resort to superior machinery to raise the water would be another vast improvement. Irrigation.

Though the soil of the district is by no means favourable to the production of cotton: yet the best varieties ought to be tried, as on account of the low temperature in the cotton season, the finer northern kinds might thrive. Cotton.

Wood is generally scarce in the district, most of it having been destroyed during the Maharatta rule; hills and valleys that were formerly wooded, are now bare of trees. The Zumeendars leave to providence the production or preservation of an occasional tree, and only the very commonest sorts are met with. This dearth of wood is injurious by preventing the erection of commodious dwellings, and rendering any little articles of furniture extremely dear. Arts requiring the consumption of wood can be little practised. Protection from the cold in the cold weather is hence also more difficult. Hence also, the coarse food of the poor inhabitants is prepared by burning cow-dung, or euphorbia stalks, the dense smoke from which flavours the food and injures the eyes. Scarcity of Wood.

Both with reference to the comforts and the arts of the inhabitants, the cultivation of trees ought to be inculcated and encouraged. The apathy of the natives, if left alone, will never effect the object. A proper proportion of forest will diminish the general temperature of the district, and especially benefit agriculture, by promoting heavy dews and rains.

The difficulties are chiefly, that natives will not go to search for young trees to plant, and that the young trees require water for a few years.

That these objections are futile, appears from the consideration that in every village the fields are here and there divided by main water-courses, never broken down, leading from the wells; and that young trees can be easily provided.

There are many valuable and useful timber trees that would thrive in the district, as I shall instance under the head of trees.

Every Zumeendar ought to be directed or requested to plant and preserve trees along the water-courses alluded to.

Ryots desirous of Improvement.

Some of the natives seem to have a taste for agricultural improvement, and in the district I have frequently seen lucerne grass well cultivated in the "khets."

At Ajmeer the government possesses a garden, which is rented for an insignificant sum to a native who retails the fruit.

Government Garden.

This garden under proper arrangements might become a source of great improvement to the district. All the best kinds of forest trees, adapted to the particular climate, could be cultivated in abundance: and any requisite quantity furnished, on demand, to the Zumeendars, who would promise to protect their subsequent growth: some of the finer and all the commoner kinds of fruit trees and flowers could also be produced for an abundant supply to the village gardens: the seeds of cotton, grasses, and trefoils, the superior kinds of grain and sugar-cane might also be furnished. I am convinced that if such a plan was to be adopted, the small present gain would be far surpassed in value by the greater prosperity of the villagers.

The Ajmeer district is generally arid, and the inhabitants are very poor and hardy: their method of cultivating is superior, especially the "jauts;" but their homes shew no comforts. At present such a people would seem to require the encouragement of a low assessment: they and their district require much fostering to promote improvement. Ryots very Poor.

At present both Zumeendars and ryots are very poor: and though the more peaceful are grateful to and satisfied with our government; yet, they often bitterly complain of their poverty, and depression: their existence is a perpetual struggle with want.

They very much complain of the "bohara" or "middle men" system. The name "bohora" is derived from "bohor" trade: the "bohoras" are generally trading brahmuns of the "paliwal" tribe, or "aswal jain seths," or "bunyas." They are quite distinct from the "bohara" tribe of Bombay and the Dukhan, who are a peculiar caste of Mussulmans. Ruinous System.

The "bohora" pays the instalments calculated on the land cultivated to the government, and advances the requisite sum for seed and food to the cultivator: in return the "bohara" receives back the whole of what he has advanced to government, and also what he has advanced to the cultivator, with interest. It appears evident that in favourable seasons, the ryot ought to benefit; however, this is seldom the case, and no doubt results from much chicanery. In an unfavourable season, all falls upon the ryot: the "bohora" having paid the land revenue to the collector, the government cannot interfere between him and the ryot: the consequence is, that the ryots' goods (bullocks, &c.) are all seized and sold, and he is ruined as much as he *can* be; while the "bohara" must thrive: the poor ryot then borrows again from the "bohora," or obtains a sum of money elsewhere, and commences "dé novo," unwilling to forsake the ground that his father tilled. Often, however, he is driven by distress and annoyance of debt, to fly for ever and forsake his home, taking refuge in some distant village.

The extortionate conduct of the "bohoras" to the ryots is notorious:—and the gross ignorance of the latter gives every facility for cheating them in their accounts: the ryots often being caused to believe twenty maunds due, when there may be only ten maunds justly claimable;—and as the "bohora" buys up the excess of grain from the ryots, in favourable seasons, at a very low price, the latter only obtains a part of what is due to him, being ignorant of the amount of balance in his favour.

Ryots cheated.

Add to all this, the fact that sometimes the sowings of one hundred have only returned fifty.

Ryost now Fewer

The assamies or ryots are on the whole at this time fewer, many having been compelled to abscond.

Content under British Rule.

The cultivators and others are quite sensible of the freedom from oppression under our rule, and are desirous to be contented. It would seem highly desirable to free them from this incubus of their old rule, the system of extortionate middle-men. The government might by proper agents advance to the assamies, at a small rate of interest, and by the same hands collect the amount of revenue when due: the cultivators being allowed to dispose of their own grain to the best advantage. A few good seasons would thus enable them to accumulate a little money, to provide against a bad season, and in the end the government would gain.

Plundering Tribes regret old times.

Many of the Rajpoots, Menas and Mairs, are dissatisfied with the British rule; looking back with regret to their own lawless, and the Maharatta times, when more was gained by highway robbery, than they now can possibly obtain by cultivating.

All, however, allow that our system of one levy of customs on the goods of traders, is just and excellent, and that the trade has greatly increased in consequence.

Istimrar Lands.

The istimrar lands, granted in perpetuity to the various thakoors, are generally deeply in pawn to the seths and "boharas:" the thakoors gain very little by their property; such is chiefly the result of their own carelessness. If the thakoors could be persuaded, it would seem a better plan, to resume some of these lands, and to pension the thakoors, liberating them from their incumbrances.

Owing to the circumstances stated, it is certain that the cultivator of Ajmeer has not benefited by coming under British rule, so much as he otherwise would have done.

Maharatta Taxes.

In addition to our own system of land tax, it seems extraordinary that in this poor district, the two most objectionable Maharatta taxes should be also still retained: these are the "fouz-kurch" from potels on "khalisa" land; and the "bhom bhao" on the "bhomias" or hereditary small land-holders: both of which are very much complained of.

Ryots pawn their Children

The ryots are occasionally so very poor, as secretly to pawn their children to the bunyas.

Fodder for Cattle.

I may here mention that fodder for cattle is generally abundant in this district. The bujra and juar stalks are cheap and very plentiful. The grasses are:

Kurrur, the best,
Sherul, good, ... } abundant after good rains.
Dhamul, good,...

Dhoop—used for horses, plentiful in low sandy soils.

Sourwul—spear grass, abundant and bad; but sometimes resorted to.

Lampas,
Gumoora, } bad; but sometimes used in scarcities.
Boor, ...

Price of Grain.

The price of the superior kinds of grain in this district is generally high. Fortunately, during the late famine in the other provinces, Ajmeer was favoured with rather a plentiful season; so that, though the price of grain rose very high, in consequence of partial exportation, still the poor were enabled to subsist in however miserable a manner. When famine does visit this district, either particularly or in conjunction with others, the most heart-rending distress occurs, and many die from starvation: at such times ties of kindred become naught: children are sold, and prostituted, for a trifle, to the more wealthy; and money, whenever possessed, will often not procure food.

On this latter point I would beg leave to make a few remarks.

Famine. In Ajmeer, and elsewhere in India, the price of corn in the towns and villages, is dependent not on the demand only, but, on the quantity of grain brought into the bazars by the bunyas, who deal in grain. On this supply, the quantity of which is daily ascertained by a chowdry in large towns, a temporary price is fixed.

The greatest quantity of corn in villages is under an embargo to the seths or "boharas," who have advanced money to the Zumeendars, who are almost all involved in debt, the poorer living literally from hand to mouth.

It is hence evident that the price of corn in the bazars is not dependent on the amount of corn in the district, but, on the speculations of the monopolizers, as to a probable rise in price.

I am quite aware that this is considered to be an equitable arrangement, on the supposed ground that the supply will always equal the demand, and that prices must find their level.

In more civilized countries this is no doubt the case: the state, when the poor complain, not interfering with the corn-factors or farmers, but having the power of acting much more effectually, by opening the ports for the importation of foreign corn, or even offering a premium on importation. Thus the holders of corn can only with profit raise the price to a certain extent; beyond which, though the government does not interfere with individuals, a public and effectual remedy is provided.

Again; in a civilized country a very small rise in the price of grain will induce the holder to sell, rather than run the risk of a fall in prices, or the ruin of the article by mildew or otherwise. In such countries the voice of the poor becomes loud in complaint, and early reaches the ears of the prince or legislature, demanding investigation or redress.

In India, when famine is actually dreaded or present, any direct interference with the monopolizers would be considered very bad political economy, on the supposition that the corn-holders *will* sell their corn, at an equitable price: and send their corn wherever the highest price can be obtained: thus, it is supposed, a certain level would result. It would, on the principle of the greatest good of the greatest number, be evidently folly to force holders to open their stores, and retail grain to the inhabitants at a certain fixed price, though even higher than ordinary; as it is evident that the neighbouring districts might be even infinitely more in want of supplies, which they would thus be prevented receiving from the more favoured one: and the corn-holders would of course be losers, by the amount of the higher price to be obtained in districts having no grain, and the favoured district could, at any rate, only suffer by an equitable recoil in the rise of price consequent on the exportation.

Were it always the case in India, that corn-holders acted on equitable principles, and could it always be insured, that in proportion to those districts in which a famine from dearth of corn exists, there would be an equal number possessing a surplus, and that this would be exported, then the equalization that would result would render interference nugatory.

But such an assumption would be incorrect.

The Governments of Europe have provided remedies. In England the importation of foreign corn is the safety valve against the distress of famine.

It is highly incumbent on every one to endeavour to provide a remedy, if possible, against famine in India: and therefore I shall offer a few remarks. Suggestions.

According to the opinions of the seths and "boharas" themselves, there is always in store three years' consumption of corn, for all Hindusthan, taking the aggregate quantities: and such was the calculation of Abul Fuzl.

To leave the regulation of the distribution of this supply to the corn-dealers or other monied men in India, will not provide against famines in certain districts at different periods.

They will not, *immediately*, receive intelligence of famine in a distant district; and when they do, however avaricious, they may have other speculations; or apathy may occasion inaction or delay.

This is proven by the fact, that while famine was raging in the "Dooab" and elsewhere, wheat and other grains were abundant and cheap to the south of the Nerbudda, while exportation was not prevented. The difficulties and expense of carriage, especially during the rains, no doubt acted as a great check in this instance, but are by no means insurmountable.

Let any impartial person examine, and he will soon be convinced that a fertile district, possessing plenty of grain, does not always export it to those districts where scarcity or famine prevails; but especially in native states, a positive prohibition is put on the exportation.

Where grain-holders determine to export grain to a famished district, they do so too slowly to provide against or remedy the evil: and this delay is augmented by the bad roads and slow carriage.

Though corn-holders or speculators *may* be tempted by a very high price, they will *wait* for one. During this delay the corn is hoarded up in the more favoured district, thus raising the price there: and the distress augments in the famished one.

During all these delays, the most dreadful misery occurs. The voice of the poor is not at first heard: they complain and murmur amongst themselves: those who have hoarded a few rupees against a rainy day, manage to exist on their little wealth; and those who have not, sell their household goods, bullocks, and wives' ornaments, for food; this is dealt out to them by the "bunyas" at a niggardly rate: at length, when means are quite exhausted, and they have waited in vain for a favourable change of the season, they abandon all hope, and the distress becomes dreadful. The relief of importing corn comes too late: many die in the mean time, and the survivors have no money to purchase grain with. The importation of corn is *only* beneficial to those who can buy it. Those relieved by charity are not a tithe of the sufferers. The inhabitants of some districts

Dreadful Distress.

habitually export corn, which is commonly produced in great excess: and yet these very districts, at times, suffer as much as poorer ones.

It would appear rational, that the money-holders in such districts, knowing that there was no corn in store, and foreseeing the near approach of scarcity, should immediately import a supply; but to trust to them would be leaning on a broken reed.

They take care to keep a sufficient supply for themselves; but profit is their object, and "who is to pay" is their inquiry. For the Government or any good pay-master, they will import; but they well know the poverty of the Zumeendars and ryots. It would seem, at first sight, that an occasional famine must put much money in the purse of the cultivators, by the great rise in price; and that the sums thus accumulated, would serve to purchase food during famines; but, let it be considered, that the profit to the cultivator is *always* small, the only benefit being to him as to others, that the cheapness of grain, when abundant crops are reaped, allows him to consume more. In a plentiful season the "boharas" or seths purchase the grain from the ryots at a cheap rate; and they are the only gainers by retailing it at an exorbitant price during famines. Thus, knowing that the ryots can not pay, the corn-holder will not send a great supply to the famished district: he will only sell corn to the "bunyas" at a very high price; and as to send any supply beyond the immediate demand would lower the price, and be against their united interest, the "bunya," therefore, will only buy of the corn-holder what he can speedily sell at a very high rate. Both parties keep up the cry of scarcity, their interest being concerned to make this appear; while in real truth, corn may be procurable in sufficient abundance for *all*, by importation; but monopolizers are prevented doing so, being aware that the poor ryot has expended or pawned his all, and cannot pay: and he may therefore die of starvation.

The equalization of the supply of corn and prices over all India, cannot be always trusted in emergencies to corn-dealers and money-holders.

But, without any infringement on the rules of political economy, a remedy can be provided; and this remedy ought to be provided by the state. It is not sufficient to sit down satisfied with raising a large subscription, or by remitting the coming revenue; for it is evident that however magnificent the subscription be, the relief must be exceedingly partial, and only extends, to those who arrive at the charitable depôts; necessarily excluding the thousands who remain in their villages to droop, or the thousands who die on the roads: and a remission of coming revenue is of no avail to the wretched utterly without present supply.

The warm feelings of sympathetic charity are gratified by beholding the joy of the thousands who may have been relieved, when departing, on the prospect of a more favourable season, to renew their labours, and again wait upon providence; but, in the glare of this noble exhibition let not the heart forget, that in proportion to every one preserved thousands have perished. Such charity is ennobling, and brings truly her own reward; but to the state must we look for a general remedy.

It does appear, to my poor idea, that in a country over the vast extent of which, a three years' consumption of grain is calculated to be the average stock in store: and in a country where famine is never universal; but, on the contrary, comparatively to the extent is very partial: and where, however difficult the roads are, no actual impediments exist, any great loss of life by famine amongst the industrious inhabitants, might be avoided: especially under a government possessing such power, such facility of information, and such accurate connexion in the various departments, regulated with wisdom, and conducted with just intentions.

The name of Acber Shah is more famous for his benevolent intentions, in preventing the effects of scarcity during famines in various provinces in India, by importing vast supples of grain from those more favoured, than for all his other achievements.

It is evident that the best remedy would be (if possible) to raise the condition of the ryot, by enabling him to reap the whole profit of his toil, after deducting the government tax; by which, in favourable seasons, he would be enabled to save sufficient money to purchase the requisite quantity of imported corn, in scarcities, for himself and family.

But, as this cannot at present be, the only other remedy, during the *actual presence* of famine, would seem to be in the coffers of the state.

The Government of course *cannot* interfere with the money or corn-holders in high-priced districts.

However extraordinary the assertion may seem, there is a very general opinion amongst the common natives, that even in the most famished districts, abundance of grain is concealed in the ground. There seems no just doubt of the fact. Such conduct may probably result from the holders' knowledge of the inability of the poor (the chief demanders) to purchase with ready money:—and they prefer that the grain should rot, rather than dispose of it, on the precarious security offered.

But, more strange still, corn has been refused at Ajmeer, during the last famine, by those who held thousands of maunds, to retail purchasers, who offered a small sum of ready money, for a very little corn, at a very high rate; even to save the demander's life.

A great cry is raised against a government forcing open the hidden garners, and justly so when considered in a civil point of view; but, suppose the fact to be proven and generally known, that a great deal of corn is concealed in a district, the property of monopolizing money-brokers, who do not exhibit any probable intention of exporting; but who pretend some speculation, while the people of the district starve: then is the government not to force the supply into the market, compelling the holders to sell at a high remunerating rate, to those who have money, and on credit to those who have none? On the principle of the preservation of the greatest number, such an interference would seem highly proper.

Although such an act would be in reality equitable; yet, on the part of any government so doing it would be highly illegal, and, as all government depends on the observance of the law, could not be wisely entered on. The principle of self-preservation and utilitarianism alike point out that the poor should not be dependent beyond a certain point on the selfish rich, for the staff of life: and the former by the law of nature would be quite authorized to resort to force, with the sole view of obtaining means for support of life, and compel the corn-holders to produce and retail the concealed corn. The poor ought not to die to satisfy the avarice of the rich. The Hindoos however want the combination requisite to compel by fear the production of the much needed supply.

There is a general belief throughout Rajwarra, that during the last dreadful famine, when thousands died of starvation, there was a great quantity of grain hidden in the country, at the very time.

The fact of finding ancient garners of corn full of grain, carbonized by time, shews that the practice of concealment is very ancient, and gives the statement every probability.

The government of India feels the greatest anxiety to protect the children of the soil; but, the wise Laws and modern instances of fire-side politicians, will not point out a way of averting famines: nor has the trust placed in the hydraulic adage of supply and price finding their own level, hitherto produced the expected result in averting famine in any degree: the supply and price being wholly dependent on the tender mercies of monopolizing speculators, solely guided by avarice.

I would wish with all deference to be permitted to suggest a remedy.

Plan Proposed.

Supposing that the quantity of grain of every kind (old and new) be ascertained in every purgunah in British India on the 1st of May and on the 1st of November every year: empower the collector in every way to obtain the necessary information, which ought to be most accurate: punish severely by fine and imprisonment any withholding of the just accounts, or peculation on the parts of native officers, or the grain-holders themselves.

Let a general return of all these reports be laid before a board by the government: and a copy of every return be speedily furnished to every magistrate in India.

Thus at one view every magistrate will perceive the relative deficiencies of supply, or the reverse, of his own and other districts, at an early period: and the nearest district having an excessive amount of grain, from which to obtain a supply.

Whenever the supply is any where too small, let the magistrate issue an "ishtihar" to the corn-brokers and bunyas, stating that, unless they immediately import the required supply of grain from other districts, so as to lower the price to the means of the poor, and proportion the supply to the consumption, the government will import what is required.

After a short time, if the corn-dealers do not give proof of having acted with energy as desired, then let the magistrate (by the aid of the H. C.'s cattle, if possible), or if not, then by hired carriage, import from the nearest most plentiful district the requisite quantity of grain: giving information, throughout his district, of the fact; and let this corn be retailed at a price just sufficient to cover the outlay, under proper agents, in quantities, from one seer to half a maund or even five maunds for bonâ fide household consumption: and on no account be allowed to be bought up by the monopolists.

The poorer sorts of natives and the common run of bunyas would come in flocks to purchase, and bless the government for the timely benevolence.

This practice being universal, the corn-monopolizers would have no inducement to keep back corn for distant speculations; but they must open their stores and reduce prices.

The magistrate would probably never need to import beyond fifteen days' consumption, as by that time the corn-dealers would be compelled either to produce supplies of grain, or lose by a total stoppage of their business.

Large quantities of grain should not be stored by the magistrate, to avoid the danger of "godown" peculation.

Diseases from bad Grain.

The grains in use in this district have not been known at any time to produce diseases, either from any quality inherent in the grain itself (such as darnel grass in Europe) or from diseases in the plant. In scarce seasons the natives have recource to the commonest and nauseous seeds that can by possibility be eaten. The seed of the common "bur" and of a small desert plant called "phog" are greedily consumed. On this diet cutaneous complaints become common; this circumstance cannot be considered to arise from any peculiar quality of the seeds; but depends on the inefficient nourishment of the system.

Under this head, I would wish shortly to allude to the extraordinary effect I have witnessed at Hoshungabad, arising from the use of new kootkie and kodhoo (two small and inferior sorts of rice), when probably diseased at particular seasons. These grains in favourable seasons become exceedingly cheap at the end of the rains: and are in general very wholesome food. It is evident that when unwholesome some peculiar disease of the plants must be the occasion: though the cause is not perceptible to the eye, like the ergot of the diseased rye.

Curious Disease.

On reaping and winnowing the crop, the whole inhabitants of a village commonly largely consume these grains as food, being very palatable. For a day or two little effect is produced: at length the whole inhabitants become maniacal, only differing in degree according to their various temperaments, the generality being "madmen gay:" all work is neglected, and the village is without regulation: this state lasts for one or two days, sometimes much longer: death occasionally occurs. The disease excited differs from Raphania, produced from eating damaged rye. Both diseases are marked by abberration of mind; but the Indian disease differs from Raphania, in making its appearance much more rapidly, and generally in the absence of convulsions, and the non-production of ulcers, and in having no permanent bad effect on the constitution. The sight of many individuals, or a whole village, labouring at once under the effects mentioned, has a very ludicrous appearance.

The roads in the district are in a great degree left to nature; but, from the dry nature of the soil, and as rain seldom falls for any long continued period, they are generally open all the year round; and in Ajmeer proper, and throughout Jodpoor and Jaepoor, the rainy season is most favourable for travellers: at the same time, the roads to the south of the Bunas, and west of the Khari-nuddee, become difficult or impracticable. Roads.

In the plains between the hills in the district, the ground is very level, and the roads are excellent; in the different passes and nullahs, the roads are very stony and difficult: it is evident that the very materials, that form the obstacle, would be the best to make good roads with. The expense would be considerable, and the inhabitants would never consent to pay.

The roads in the district are sufficiently good, and seldom or never are so obstructed as to interfere with the comforts of the inhabitants or impede the trade.

A very good road has been made, and is kept up by the superintendent Mr. Macnaghten, from Ajmeer over the Ana-sagur ghaut to the foot of the pass leading to Poshkur: another road has also been made over the Kishengurh pass, by the same gentleman, and is a good and very useful one. Part of the road to Nusseerabad, three miles in extent through the pass, is artificial, and has lately been improved and rendered capable for wheel carriages, by a shorter cut. A carriage road has also been cut through the hills to Poshkur, by Mr. Macnaghten.

The number of the inhabitants as taken at the last census, has been already given. At present it is a general opinion that the poorer classes, especially the cultivators, have owing to distress, diminished in numbers since the British Population.

rule: and that traders and bankers originally of the district, as well as those from other neighbouring districts who sought refuge at Ajmeer, have increased and still continue increasing in numbers, and vastly in wealth. It is to be regretted that this beneficent result of good government should not also have become manifest in the state of the far more numerous cultivators.

The population is divided into classes, as follows:

Brahmuns.

The Chinnayut brahmuns are the purohits or household priests of Ajmeer: they are divided into six tribes; the Gour, the Goozur-gour, the Diva, the Surasoot, the Sikawar and Parik; they all can eat and drink together; they came originally from Hurreeana.

The Goozurattee brahmuns.

The Pokhurna brahmuns; said to have been beldars, who dug out Poshkur lake, and in consequence were created brahmuns: they still worship the kodhalie or pickaxe at the dusseerah: they are most numerous at Pokhurn in Marwar.

The Sreemalee brahmuns; equivalent to the dhooby brahmuns.

The Nundwana and Paliwal brahmuns; are traders; were formerly located at Nundwana and Pali, and were then chiefly robbers, conducting their excursions on horseback: they subsequently became traders: they are said still to worship a bridle on the dusseerah, in memory of their former state. They now are principally the "boharas" or "middle-men" between the government and the cultivators, eating up all the latter's gains. They are also very widely spread as "boharas" in India.

Shewug brahmuns; these always conduct the worship of temples. Poshkurna brahmuns; another division.

Ducôt and Boora brahmuns; these are beggars; they arose from a mixture of brahmun and aheer blood: the first sort will take articles in charity that a pure brahmun will not so receive, such as oil, &c.: the second sort "wait on dying men's shoes," and claim the apparel the rich die in: they are the terror of fat bunyas, especially if met with early in the morning.

Rajpoots.

The Chutrees or Rajpoots are—

The Chohan and the Rhatore; conquerors at former periods: now the most numerous.

The Gôr are of very ancient date.

The Gôrawattie and the Surwur are peculiar to this district.

The Cuchwaha, the Sankla, the Seesodiya, and the Burgoozur; these are few in numbers and scattered.

The Purihar, now few, were the first who conquered the country from the "Meenas" and "Mairs."

Byess or Trading Division.

The Aswal or Serawuck tribe, of the Seetumber division of the "Jain" sect were Rajpoots, originally of Oswa in Marwar, and were converted by a saint to the "Jain" faith: they worship images of the "Owtars" or incarnations of Parswa Nath: their present and last "Owtar" is the thirty-third in number, and occurred in the person of Bhachurad, a "Pramara" Rajpoot of the "Soda" tribe, who appeared at Parkur, where the most sacred image now is, in the possession of a small body of "Soda" Rajpoots, and the pilgrimage to worship which image, is resorted to at a great expense. This image is so sacred as to be buried in the sand with great secrecy, and is annually dug up for the occasion. The Oswals are an exceedingly wealthy body of men, and are widely scattered all over India. In Ajmeer they are numerous. They all, more or less, possess the peculiar "Tatar" expression of features.

The Suraogee tribe, of the Degumber division of the "Jain" faith, are similar in habits and wealth, and appearance to the Oswal tribe. Both have priests of their own body, termed "jetties," who are supposed to be exceedingly learned in the voluminous works of Jain, their founder, containing as they suppose, every science: they act as medical as well as spriritual attendants. These "Jetties" have a bad name, being much given to intrigue, and supposed to be equally alert to poison as to cure.

The tenets of these people, are deistical: their habits less *really* humane, than humane to a false and merely ceremonious extent, especially in the impossible protection, which they pretend to extend to insects even of filthy kinds. Though aware that at every step they must tread upon numerous insects, they will yet interfere to prevent the koomars making and burning earthern pots in the rains, because insects then abound, and would be killed by the smoke and fire: and this interference, to the inconvenience of the other inhabitants.

Their tenets inculcate that they should never possess more than is actually sufficient; yet, they not only accumulate millions, but do so chiefly by sub-renting provinces of native states; and by buying and hoarding up vast quantities of corn, raising the price in famines, often to a great extent, rendering it impossible for the poor to buy, who may therefore die: this conduct the Oswals and Suraogees reconcile to their consciences, though they will not swallow a gnat or kill a vile insect.

The Jetties and brahmuns were, even as late as Ackber Shah's time, deadly enemies: now, they are on very friendly terms.

The Oswals and Suraogees also allow a class of female devotees: who are often seen at Ajmeer going about in dirty cotton garments with a dirty cloth over their mouths, suspended under the nose, to prevent any insect entering the mouth.

Maiserie, Uggur Wallah, and Khutree, bunyas; are of brahminical faith: the first act as "boharas" also; the others are general traders.

Ghundee; perfumers or uttars; generally in that trade.

Bunyas of numerous tribes.

SOODRA, OR WORKING DIVISION.

Bunyas; some are of Soodra caste.

Kayets; writers.

Thailies; oilmen.

Jauts; cultivators.

Aheers; cowherds, also cultivators.

Kuhars, of the better sort are also Soodra caste.

The class of artificers was formerly of this division, and as society increased became absolutely necessary: the class became, therefore, separated from the Soodra, under the head of the "athara pon" or eighteen divisions.

The "athara pon" no longer pure Soodras, are again subdivided into different degrees of purity, as follows; outum, mudhim, and adhim.

Durzees; tailors.

Malees; gardeners.

Khaties; carpenters.

Mochees; saddlers and fine leather-workers.

Tumboolis; pawn cultivators.

Chitrams; portrait painters.

Koomars; potters.

Thatheras and kuseras; the one braziers, the other brass founders.

Sonars; goldsmiths.

Rungkar or rungsaj; dyers and painters.

Dhobys; washermen.

Bulahies; weavers, and used as guides or doreehas, and as "beegaries" or pressed porters, from time immemorial.

Dheemurs; fishermen, and often bearers.

Kasids or "gutchkas:" messengers or expresses.

Dujas or "nishan burdars;" standard-bearers.

Munnee-karuks; jewel cutters.

Kories or kolis; weavers or porters, and workmen generally.

Raj; mason.

Below these and removed entirely from the Soodra, are the "untez;"

Kunjurs; gipsies, who eat reptiles of all kinds.

Dhôms; eat carrion.

Rewarries; camelmen.

Kharols; salt and saltpetre makers.

Churuns and bhats; bards.

Churun-kal-mochies; shoe-makers.

Kutiks, chumars, and raeghurs; curriers and skinners; the kutiks will only prepare goat skins, which they dye red; the chumars and raeghurs will both prepare the skins, and eat the carrion bodies of cows, &c.

Bheels and meenas, of hilly districts; mairs, of Mairwarra; kolie, of Ramghur and Goozurat; aborigines.

Below these again are the "mileetch" or outcastes;

Thorie and Mihtur; Hindoos, perform any filthy offices.

Bhungie; half Hindoo, half Mussulman; perform same offices.

The Muhommedans are chiefly numerous at Ajmeer and in its vicinity.

Sheik, Pathân, Mogul and Syud; at and near Ajmeer.

Cheeta; converted mairs and meenas.

Of the population the most influential and respectable are the seths and sahookars of the different Byess tribes. Many have found protection and augmented wealth under the British rule: and they very generally appreciate the advantage of our government.

Most of the seths who reside at Ajmeer are very wealthy and do not enter into trade.

Fine Buildings. The number of very wealthy natives and costly buildings at Ajmeer indicate rather a forced state of prosperity, many of the seths being partial refugees from neighbouring states and having been induced to erect splendid residences, by the energetic instigation of the British Superintendents, anxious for the welfare of Ajmeer. The seths themselves state that in the event of a proper settlement being made by our government in Marwar, many wealthy natives will return again to their original homes, and that although they might keep up their houses at, still their wealth would in the main, be lost to, Ajmeer.

At first, speculation in opium was eagerly entered upon, especially in Mr. Wilder's time: however, as loss often resulted, this gambling trade has been now nearly altogether abandoned. *Opium Speculation*

The seths state that they would be better satisfied with a fixed order, being placed under the regulations, as at Agra, from which there could be no departure, especially, as under a succession of superintendents very different views may be acted upon. *Regulations Desired.*

The sahookars complain very much that our government will in no way assist them in obtaining redress in neighbouring native states, where often large sums due to them are unjustly detained, and their connexions maltreated. Generally those who detain the money due, are secretly protected by the native state, and it is in vain for the Ajmeer sahookar to complain in that quarter, unless he resorts to ruinous bribery. *Redress from Native States desired.*

The cultivators, the most numerous class of all, are by far the most wretched, and the most worthy of the British protection. They are far too highly assessed for the nature of the soil and climate, and can never much benefit even in the best seasons, owing to the remorseless avarice of the "boharas." *Ryots most worthy of protection.*

If the assessment was properly proportioned, and the government appointed agents to advance the requisite sum to the ryots, at a moderate interest, and to collect the revenue *after* the crops should be reaped, and proceeds realized, then the ryots would become thriving, numerous and happy.

This district, naturally very poor, is much oppressed by the numbers of religious mendicants who force a livelihood from the superstition of the ignorant inhabitants. They are nagas, gosains, naths or jogis, bhats, charuns, byragies, sunjogies, in great numbers, and all prey on this poor district. *Religious Mendicants.*

If the different tribes of these idle people were placed under darogahs chosen from their own body, and granted land now uncultivated, being forbidden to beg under a penalty, a most advantageous result would be produced:

and highly intelligent natives assert that the tribes in question would not object to the change.

Pressed Porters. Of the poorer classes of the villagers, the bulahie, the chumar, the raeghur and the korie, are and have been pressed from time immemorial as guides and porters from village to village, for all travellers; and they are granted privileges in consequence, of all dead animals' skins, and of a certain quantity of land.

A great cry has been raised against this system of "beegarie kam;" but, the people themselves infinitely prefer conveying the goods of travellers from village to village, and being there exchanged and allowed at once to return, to being paid two or three annas for the whole march of four or five coss. Unless the hardship is explained to the natives in question, they are too much habituated to it to perceive it.

In other parts of the country, where the hardship has been explained, these people have become very extortionate.

Habits. The habits of the people, except the upper ranks, are not very cleanly; owing to poverty, the cold of the winter, and the general use of opium.

Dwellings. In the city of Ajmeer are the best dwellings, some of the houses of the most wealthy seths being very extensive; one or two lately erected have cost two or three lakhs of rupees, and form imposing objects even from the outside of the city walls. The streets of Ajmeer are, some wide and handsome, but the generality narrow: they are often very much wanting in cleanliness, though in this respect, very much superior to the towns of native states. On the whole the buildings of the poorer sorts are more commodious than those ordinarily met with elsewhere.

Ancient Buildings. The most ancient building is beyond the city wall, under Taraghur, called the "arahie din ka jhompra," a Jain temple traditionally said to have been erected by spirits in two days and a half, and hence the name. The building must, when complete, have been very extensive: the remains have still a very elegant appearance, from the number, the height, and lozenged carving of the columns which support the dome. The whole is built of yellow soft fine-grained sandstone from Marwar. The Mahommedans at an early period dismantled the greatest part of this temple: and converted what still remains into a mosque. At the period that this temple was erected, the Jain faith and rule were probably paramount in the northwest of India. There appears to be no trace of the date. Most probably this temple was erected at the same period with the other "takshac" monuments scattered over Sinde and Rajwarra, especially those at Cheetore and Komulmēr.

The other chief building is the durgah of Kwaja Moyen-ud-deen, formerly spoken of.

The government magazine is formed partly of, and on the site of, an ancient palace of Acber Shah. The powder magazine containing a large quantity of gunpowder, has no lightning conductor. On one occasion the electric fluid struck very near the powder magazine. The most awful consequences would necessarily result from the explosion of such a large quantity of gunpowder, especially on account of the close proximity to the town. Magazine.

Conductors, sufficient in number, and properly erected, would obviate this danger. I heard it stated, as a reason for the non-erection of conducting rods, that they were supposed to increase the danger. Such result could only arise from imperfect insulation of the rods: which circumstance on one occasion caused the conflagration of Lord Grosvenor's house in London. Lightning Conductors.

In the villages the houses are built of mud, and generally have a small yard surrounded by a mud wall, in the form of a cul-de-sac, to contain cattle, &c. at night: the roofs are flat, of well beaten mud, mixed with chopped straw and pebbles: these if taken care of are very lasting, as the duration of rain is seldom beyond two or three days, with dry intervals. The great scarcity of wood and canes prevents the use of thatched roofs, which would certainly be much cooler. The villages are generally erected on slight elevations, more in former reference to defence, than to Village Houses.

avoid water lodging: this elevation, and the nature of the soil and rainy season, render the villages dry. The houses are sufficiently commodious for the inhabitants. So scarce is wood, that the supports for the flat mud roofs are obliged generally to be made of the stems of the asclepias gigantea or mudar plant, laid closely together. These mud dwellings are plastered with yellow or white earth, and look rather clean and well, even when closely inspected. The inhabitants do not seem, in general, crowded. Forage is not allowed to waste, and the dung of the cattle is used for fuel: all ashes and filth and old straw, &c., are accumulated outside the towns for manure: hence the narrow passages between the houses are generally clear of decomposing dirt.

Sites of Villages.

I think the construction and situation of the villages in this disrict, exhibit no causes conducive to unhealthiness.

Bedding.

The beds do not differ from those of other parts of India. All who can afford to do so have charpaies to sleep upon, which elevate the sleeper one foot and a half above the ground. The natives when the weather is dry and warm, sleep on the roofs of their houses, or in small upper stories in the hot season and intervals of the rains. This with the general elevation of the villages above the plains, serves to protect the inhabitants very much from the effects of any floating febrile miasmata. The scarcity of wood puts it out of the power of many to possess beds: and those who have them, keep them till very old and filthy. The vermin are complained of as a great cause of discomfort. On the death of one of superior caste, the defunct's bed and bedding are burnt or thrown away: and no respectable person will receive either. The bedding is very simple, consisting of the clothes worn in the day, and a quilt to those who can afford one.

Clothing.

In the hot season the clothing is worn the same as elsewhere in India; but, in the cold season, quilted garments are necessarily much worn by those who can afford them. These are hoarded up with care by the poor, till from long use, they often become very filthy, and would certainly tend much to spread infection, or propagate any cutaneous or other contagious diseases. The great poverty of the poor prevents the change of garments sufficiently often. Sheep are fortunately numerous, and wool therefore cheap: coarse blankets are very common and low-priced, and felts of coarse wool, beat into the shape of a short cloak, with a hood for the head, called "numda," are cheap and very much used in the rains, effectually protecting from the wet. The natives' garments are seldom clean, either those of the women or the men. Poverty and the cold of winter foster these habits of dirt; but, this state also much results from the general use of opium, or other intoxicating drugs. A man under the influence of opium cares little for any thing in this world.

On festive occasions the garments of the women and the turbans of the men are peculiarly gay, being coloured most brilliantly; the dyes being of very beautiful though evanescent colours. This gay appearance forms a strong contrast with their usual state. That an occasional very brilliant exterior marks the slattern, is quite illustrated in this district.

Calicoes and chintzes of English manufacture, and also flannel and coarse woollen cloths, are much higher appreciated than Indian articles, and are worn by all who can afford to purchase them.

The furniture is of the coarsest and simplest description: and is scarce even of this kind, almost the only articles being beds, and a few low wooden seats in some large houses. The superior classes of Rajpoots use our chairs and tables when to be had, especially on ceremonious occasions of visits from the British. Furniture

As previously remarked, fuel is very scarce: the smoke of the dry dung and "thuar" stalks, and of the "salar" and "gugal" woods, which are most commonly used, is very injurious to the eyes. Fuel.

The diet consists of the cheapest grains, sometimes of very inferior quality. Wheat would no doubt be used by all could they afford to do so. Barley is next in request. Juar and bujra come after barley in point of demand; and Diet.

they form with maize the staple diet of the poorer. To those accustomed to wheat, the latter mentioned grains are very intolerable as a permanent article of diet: and for a long time strangers do not become reconciled to it. On the other hand, those who have been long habituated to this diet, very much prefer it.

Marwar sends out artisans all over India, especially "sonars," and I have heard these people at a great distance from Marwar, regret the "bujra rotie" with much feeling; like that of the Scots respecting oatmeal.

Moong ka dal is the legume most preferred; but, "moth ka dal" is commonly used by the poorer: the latter is harder and often a little bitter. Dal of some kind is an absolute necessary for the poor, without which, the dry, hard, tasteless "bujra" or other cakes are with difficulty swallowed even with hunger as sauce.

Vegetables are scarce and much sought after: every edible weed is consumed as "greens," and the young pods of the "khejra" (mimosa edibilis) are a great blessing to the poorer, by whom they are largely consumed: the pods are preserved dried in earthen pots. Tamarinds where procurable are much used as a zest; or a lime with mint and ginger.

Ghee is used by all who can afford it; and oil of mustard by those who cannot: the very poorest consume "rookhie rotie" (flour and water baked) a very wretched diet.

In famines the seeds of "phog" and "bruit" are eagerly resorted to: it is difficult to conceive how any one can manage to swallow the flour of these seeds. Dried jujubes ("bier") yield a flour used at all seasons called "birchan," that is very palatable, and generally procurable every where.

On this generally poor diet, which the commonalty can only sparingly consume, their appearance is muscular, slender, and they are active. They are generally tall and personally powerful people. They are more patient in their poor diet, and their stomachs crave less, by the moderate use of opium. The higher classes of Rajpoots and others live very well, and often luxuriously. By Rajpoots, meat and fish are eaten; the wild hog being especially prized.

Some seths actually feed their cows and buffaloes on raisins, almonds, and pistachio nuts, and then drink the milk as soon as enough has been secreted, imagining that the milk is very nourishing.

On the whole, the diet of the poor, though stinted is not productive of disease, except in those cases, where the most inferior kind is long used, in insufficient quantity, when cutaneous disorders of a scabrous kind appear.

Water is almost always sufficient in quantity for the consumption of the people; but, generally of bad quality, as before described. From the use of this water, dracunculus or guineaworm, is very commonly met with among the people both rich and poor. Diarrhœa and dyspepsia are also the effects of the use of bad and alkaline waters.

Employments.

The employments are almost exclusively of an agricultural nature; and as this district is exceedingly poor in that respect, the circumstance is to be the more regretted. It is to be regretted that the energies of the people cannot be roused and directed to manufactures in the larger villages and towns; as they would then not be solely dependent on the crops.

Manufactures required

Large capital would of course be required to establish manufactures, and it is a great pity that the enormously wealthy seths will not so employ their hoards.

The woollen manufacture on an extensive scale, might become exceedingly beneficial to this district.

Wool.

Wool of a very superior quality is produced by the sheep of Jessulmeer: and the same breed of sheep would very probably thrive well in Ajmeer, the pasturage being very dry and abundant. These sheep might find food on, and occupy the numerous waste lands and hills in the district. In a few years the produce of wool would be great, and from it cloth might be manufactured of a quality sufficiently good for ordinary purposes; the whole of the H. Co.'s troops might be supplied with cloth for clothing, and that far superior to that which is now distributed to them. Such a manufacture would necessarily employ a great many hands, and indigo (either wild or cultivated) would by coming into demand, yield further occupation.

Dyes. The red dyes of "al," "majith" and "lac" are abundantly produced in the neighbouring states, and would yield good and cheap dyes, also affording much occupation.

The finer kind of blankets, such as are now made at Jessulmeer, would be an article of great demand, if manufactured at a cheaper rate at Ajmeer.

Sheep Farms. The establishment of sheep farms for wool, and of woollen cloth manufactures, would be great blessings to this district. The capital, the article, and the workmen are present; but the directing hand and energy are wanting.

Lead Mine. The only present employment that might be deleterious to health, is that of the Ajmeer lead mine; but I have never heard that the Assamies so engaged suffer from the colic common to people so employed.

Customs. The customs of the people in relation to the different castes are much the same here as elsewhere in India. Except amongst the hard-working agriculturists, there is a greater disposition to idleness than elsewhere. The number of holidays observed is very great, both those of Hindoos and of Mahommedans, being mutually celebrated: this is especially the case in cities. These frivolous ceremonies are a great interruption to business of any kind: and of course, serve to prejudice the mind against application of any sort, especially if of a new and difficult nature. At the great fairs the trading classes combine pleasure with profit.

Necessity makes the agriculturists work hard; but the whole people, and above all the Rajpoots, are yet by disposition idly inclined: and nowhere is the "dolce far niente" principle more highly appreciated.

Laws. The general protection afforded, causes the generality to acknowledge the benefit of the administration of our laws; but, among the Rajpoots, Mairs, and Meenas, the recollection of their predatory habits still exists: and no doubt many would be glad again to abandon their sterile fields, and resort to highway robbery, as one successful "*rade*" might supply them with food for a year: and they would willingly run the risk of being occasionally robbed in return as often happened in former times. Fear of prompt punishment alone makes them respect the British laws of "meum and tuum." In reality they are still quite of Rob Roy's opinion. However; as it is very much to be doubted whether the general protection of property, even in the most civilized states, is not infinitely more dependent on fear of the penalties of the laws, than on innate principles of honesty or virtue resulting from education, in the great mass of the people; the Rajpoots and Meenas are not so much to be condemned as the insufficient power of the laws to restrain them.

In *time,* industry might become loved for herself, and the wealth she creates.

Erroneous Opinion of Rajpoot Character.

I have frequently heard lamented, what is called the depressed state of the Rajpoot: his sword being useless, and his martial character depreciated; but, to convert his sword into a ploughshare, is ultimately to benefit the body at large, and to make the Rajpoot a more useful individual; though a long time will elapse e'er some of the tribes will become active and willing tillers of the ground.

Let any one reflect on the immense improvement of the highlands of Scotland, from what they were before civilization was almost forced upon them. The measures to produce the effect were no doubt severe, and caused great discontent; but the result is excellent, and favourably estimated by almost all the highlanders themselves.

A similar result may be hoped for in the district of Ajmeer, especially under vigilant superintendence, and on making the assessment proportionate to the crops, to be levied by trust-worthy agents.

The warlike character of the Rajpoot, has, I think, been very much over-rated. There appears to be very little chivalrous feeling in his breast. By nature Rajpoots are generally powerful muscular men: active by habit, and practising gymnastics, (though when not excited, inclined to indolence in a high degree :) those who possess horses are generally good horsemen. Some are by constant practice dexterous in the use of lance or sword: and individually must be often superior to one of an enemy trained to act in combination, according to a rigid system of discipline. But, amongst a large body of Rajpoot horse, only a few would be found such superior men at arms, or so to venture. The Rajpoots do not possess the cool deliberate courage ready to dare any danger, and requiring no artificial excitement. According to their own accounts even, in their former attacks on caravans or towns, surprise was their object, and if successful, they were equally cruel and rapacious, shewing no mercy to their captives : and if they met with much resistance, became as cowardly as they had before been violent, and resorted to flight; fighting was not their object. In all their single combats and all assaults, they resorted to the excitement of opium, e'er commencing battle; their own bards describe the eyes of the heroes as being red from opium. Among their rajahs the treacherous murders of each other, on record, were numerous, and long premeditated : as for instance, the murder of the Rana of Odeypoor, near Kotah. In the defence of towns or forts by Rajpoots the occasional performance of the ceremony of "johur" has been lauded as heroic though terrible: this has, however, been most falsely estimated. The immolation was never performed with the stern philosophy of a Spartan. On perceiving that they could hold out no longer, the Rajpoots determined on the death of their women and children, rather than allow them to fall into the hands of the enemy. Savage jealousy and opium together excited them to perform the "johur," and after the murder of all they held dear, the Rajpoot men, then taking more opium, and clothed in yellow garments, rushed un-reflectingly on the foe, to receive their deaths, dealing at the same time as many as they could to the enemy. Acting in this way was surely not indicative of a pure and noble courage. What can be said of a man, to whom a high state of intoxication is requisite to make him fight? Or, supposing the words gin or brandy to be substituted for opium, then how would the Rajpoot's performance of "johur" be estimated?

The habitual use of intoxicating drugs is constant amongst all classes in this district; from simple tobacco, to the coveted opium. Intoxicating Drugs

Tobacco seems in no way injurious to any. Bhang and ganja, if consumed in large quantities habitually, are very injurious, suspending the powers of the mind during the period of greatest effect, and occasioning a state of permanent fatuity, more or less partial; at length the body also dwindles away, from insufficient nourishment, appetite being much impaired, owing to the dyspeptic state that always accompanies the habitual use of the drug. Tobacco.

The "churrus" or resin of bhang, either the natural exudation, or artificially extracted from the cannabis sativa, is more injurious to the constitution, than the plant itself. Hemp.

Distilled spirits, if used in moderation, do not appear to act injuriously on the consumers. Spirits are secretly used in large quantities, by the superior classes of natives. Alcohol is the really exciting ingredient; but, to enhance the price, the most incongruous and absurd materials are mixed. Spirits.

Opium, when attainable, is used by a large portion of the people: especially Rajpoots, Meenas and Mairs. The quantity consumed by individuals is often very great. I have made on this point every inquiry, and it appears that decidedly dangerous effects to the body from the excessive use, are very rare. Where injury does result, a state of dyspepsia first appears, with obstinate constipation, the body wastes away gradually: after a few years, diarrhœa supervenes, much undigested food being passed; this diarrhœa seems to depend on partial paralysis of the sphincters, and muscular tissue of the intestines: great emaciation and general paralysis precede death. Another class suffers in early youth from the use of opium; a state of satyriasis being produced that, by indulgence, gives rise to excessive emaciation and death. Opium.

The very large portion of those who use opium habitually and largely, do not suffer at all in the body. On the contrary, they are less liable to fever or rheumatism: their consumption of food is more moderate, the appetite being less keen: and they seem really to be less liable to the ills that flesh is heir to. In very numerous instances, they attain to old age of a hale nature.

The quantity of opium used daily by individuals, becomes at length very great; but, as in the use of alcoholic fluids, so, in the use of opium, there is a period up to which the dose must be gradually augmented to an acme; and beyond this, must be again diminished in quantity by the consumer, the same effects resulting still.

Effect on the mind.

The effect of the use of opium on the minds of those habitually taking it is very deleterious. The takers of large doses become perfectly useless to themselves and others, during their own happy or terrible dreams. All are rendered less useful members of society: the indolent naturally become quite inert; and those who must work, do so with far less spirit and energy, than they otherwise would. The intoxication from opium affords the most ridiculous states for observation. I have seen a mussalchee running before an elephant at night, repeatedly set fire to his dhotie; and a Rajpoot lolling back with his tongue out covered with flies.

The very stupifying effects of opium render its habitual use among a people more injurious to them, than the use of alcoholic beverages; but the opium is not more (if even so much) injurious to the health.

Those who rejoice at the stoppage of the opium trade to China, on moral grounds, do not perhaps reflect, that a people disposed to such artificial excitement, will (if in the kingdom of nature) find a worse substitute.

The use of opium in various forms is becoming very general, in both England and France, as a stimulant to salacity, and a temporary subduer of care. It has been habitually used in England and Scotland to a very great extent in well known cases, with even beneficial effects. One was the instance of a lady of rank, who from long use took her laudanum in tea-cupsful, with great relief to the rheumatic pains she suffered under, and who lived to a great age. Another lady had long laboured under gastrodynia, and she at length took with relief, to the extent of a large table spoonful of the best Turkey opium ground in water.

Amongst the cases related in Christison's Toxicology, are two very remarkable ones; first, the Earl of Mar had taken two or three ounces of laudanum daily for nearly thirty years, without any injurious effects; but, with relief to the pain endured; his mind remained clear, and he entered society as usual. Second, an eminent literary character who died at the age of 63, had since the age of 15 taken opium to excess: for many of his latter years, his daily dose was a quart of three parts laudanum, and one part alcohol, with no injurious effects. These cases are only an iota in comparison to the thousands of instances that have probably been concealed.

In relation to the political economy, opium eating is more to be condemned than the use of spirits. An opium eater will cultivate less land than a spirit drinker, and that much unwillingly and the soil for the poppy must be of the very best description; and as opium when a sale is found for it, yields more profit than wheat, the latter cultivation is in consequence neglected, the price of grain rises, and there is less provision against famine.

Koot formerly used.

Formerly, when opium was not produced in Rajwarra, the inhabitants largely consumed the root of the costus arabicus ("koot") which was smoked as a stimulant. This root is also said to have been largely exported to China.

All classes use Stimulants.

In general, every class of natives here, from the brahmun to the bhungie, resort to some stimulant habitually; the higher castes secretly. This is well known to be the case: and it is probably owing to this, that even the most respectable natives, seeing the constant use of wine and beer at the tables of Europeans, openly express their conviction, that the latter are courageous or fight our battles solely by the stimulus of drink: they will not believe that the use of spirits or wine on the field of battle would be considered disgraceful and meet with punishment due to cowards; but they declare their conviction, that the "sahib log shurab ke jor se lurte!"

Rajpoots under Stimulus. When religious prejudice had united the Rajpoots at former periods, they offered a most obstinate resistance against their Mahommedan invaders; and hence arose the lamentation of the emperor Humaiyoon, "that such a handful of sand should have caused the loss of so much Islamite blood."

Morals. The people of this district are not a moral race: their morals are now, however, undergoing a certain degree of cultivation; but the far greater portion act morally on compulsion, and not by conviction.

Education. The generality are quite without education. Brahmuns, bunyas, and seths are the educated classes. Their education extends to reading, writing and casting accounts in a simple manner. The most learned brahmuns are only very superficially acquainted with their own "pooranas," and their more modern doctrines of sects. The same may be said of the "jetty" priests of the Jain faith. Amongst the superior classes of Mahommedans at Ajmeer, a certain knowledge of Oordoo and Persian reading and writing is attained: just sufficient to enable the parties to act respectably as vakeels or office employès. The Mahommedans generally obtained this degree of lore at Delhie.

At Ajmeer, there are numerous brahmun and jetty teachers; and in general every large village possesses an "oostad" or teacher. Those taught by brahmuns lay great stress on the acquirement by rote of Sanscrit "ashloks" from the shastras, the meaning of which is very seldom understood by the boys, but the sound takes a firm hold of the memory.

A love of literature has certainly not hitherto in any instance appeared.

The prospect of profitable employment will alone induce the parents of youths to allow their children to study long enough to gain a really useful degree of knowledge.

The Government has twice established an English school

at Ajmeer. The first attempt failed: and the school was judiciously abolished by Lord W. Bentinck. An English school was again established in 1836, on a more extensive and expensive scale. A favourable result remains as yet a desideratum. The greater part of the scholars after attaining a moderate knowledge of reading, writing and arithmetic in the vernacular, would be immediately withdrawn from the school by the parents, who consider such acquirements sufficient: and the most soothing arts require to be employed by the master, pundits, and moonshees, to induce the parents to allow their children to remain and prosecute the study of English: and this consent is only extorted on the confident prospect of future employ, held out.

Should many learned scholars result, the expectations of the greater number must be disappointed.

In the large number of scholars in the Ajmeer school, six or seven may read the tasks they have learned with tolerable fluency: not one can however be considered even a moderate English scholar, and by far the greater number are very young, and slowly progress in learning their own native reading and accounts.

The results of this and the other schools in India, except in the Calcutta Medical College, are very discouraging: the number of scholars annually brought forward, completed to a degree of practical usefulness, is indeed very small; the general amount of acquirement is in no way equivalent to the expenditure and labour bestowed.

The system appears wrong: a degree of energy is required to superintend, that shall not rest satisfied with the partial results that native indolence alone will yield, and a degree of honesty that shall not endeavour to blind the Government with got-up "flash" examinations.

If the Government call for a return, shewing the annual expense of each institution in India; the number of complete scholars annually turned off; the number of years that each scholar has taken in completing himself; and the annual expense per head for every scholar in the schools, then the true state of the case would be seen.

Ajmeer Government School. The annual expense of the Ajmeer school is five thousand and fifty-two Company's Rupees.

The number of scholars varies, but averages one hundred and fifty per mensem.

The cost per annum to Government, for each scholar (most of whom are little boys learning vernacular), thirty-three Company's Rupees.

The number of perfect English scholars is an absolute blank.

The number of tolerable English scholars is about six.

The remainder are the very young, learning the mere elements of English, Oordoo, or Hindusthani.

The attendance at the school averages about seven hours per diem, *for half the year;* taking into consideration, the great number of holidays, and the number of scholars daily absent.

This school has cost the Government about twenty thousand Company's Rupees, since the re-establishment: and *not one* scholar has been produced fit for office employment, although those, now the best, entered the school nearly as much advanced as they are at present.

Any farther remarks on this subject would be out of place here.

Mode of rearing Children. The children are reared in the usual hardy way.

Police. The number of police, and the irregular horse at the immediate disposal of the Ajmeer magistrate, is barely sufficient for the most ordinary occasions, even at the city. For any extra occasion a sufficient force does not exist.

Bodies of armed marauders, of thirty or more in numbers, mounted and with loaded matchlocks, sometimes cross the country, robbing unresisted where they please.

Three or four suwars and half a dozen chapprasies at the head village of the Purgunnah, can be of no use in such cases; except to convey to the magistrate the intelligence that the country *has been* infested by robbers, or robbed: by which time the marauders "non sunt inventi."

The villagers, on such occurrences, naturally complain very loudly of want of proper protection.

Those who are of the same clans as the marauders, state that a body of forty or fifty mounted police would effectually protect the district: especially, if well commanded, and raised among the very people who are now inclined to be the robbers. By stationing, in different parties, such a police on various roads leading from Marwar, the inroads of robbers would be early known, and could then be provided against at once. The influence of the mounted police, so constituted, would be great in deterring by fear or persuasion their old companions.

The police of the city of Ajmeer is generally vigilant and sufficient for protection.

City Police.

The attention of the police is also directed to preserving the city in as cleanly a state, as the means at the disposal of the cotwal will allow.

Human ordure and other filth in the by-streets, constitute a nuisance that ought to be removed, as likely to be injurious to the health of the inhabitants, especially during the too frequent and fatal prevalence of the small-pox. This state might be remedied by the levy of a small poll-tax on the inhabitants; regulated according to the wealth or poverty of individuals; and with the proceeds constantly employing a sufficient number of scavengers, in keeping the lanes and streets scrupulously clean.

The inhabitants will never of themselves make any such regulations.

The city is very well drained, naturally, owing to its situation: in heavy rain the water runs off through some of the streets in rapid torrents.

Jail.

The jail is situated in an old patched up Mahommedan building, a few hundred yards from the town walls. It is separated entirely from other buildings, and is in a very airy and dry situation. The accommodation for the prisoners is sufficient in space. The security of the place against escape may be doubted; supposing the prisoners unite in an effort to do so, the walls being low, and the burkundaz guard small.

Jail Hospital. The hospital is hardly worthy of the name, being an arched stone-shed in one of the angles: small, but, sufficient for the average number of sick; protection from the sun and rain is afforded, but the ventilation is insufficient. The greatest disadvantage of this hospital is, that being situated without the quadrangle, within which the prisoners are chained and guarded at night, and owing to there being no spare burkundazes, the sick, however ill they may be, or however infectious their complaints, are obliged to be removed within the quadrangle and placed amongst the healthy prisoners: an arrangement mutually inconvenient and often very cruel.

Indeed it is evident, that a more absurd practice could not exist.

Fortunately the climate is exceedingly healthy: the number of sick in jail very small: mortality very rare.

Number of Prisoners. The average monthly number of prisoners is about one hundred and fifty. The prisoners are generally muscular and powerful men, of marauding tribes. Previously led to commit crime for the support of life, rather than work or beg; they soon become reconciled to the confinement, during which they are well fed and not worked to an extent deserving the name.

It is notorious that most prisoners of these tribes, come in somewhat emaciated; but, in the course of six months, they become very stout and robust.

The prisoners are generally dirty in their persons: only those who choose performing regular ablutions.

A certain number of prisoners proceed every morning, except upon Sundays, to work on the roads or elsewhere; they are led at a slow rate to the scene of action: by the time they arrive it is nearly time to return, a very little work is done, and the prisoners march back again.

The new system of giving the prisoners rations would be an excellent one, if it could be properly acted on; but, every prisoner who pleases, does now and always will continue to, exchange some of his provisions, with the bunya or others for opium, or whatever his favourite stimulant may be. Thus the prisoner manages to pass a happy dreamy existence during his captivity.

This objectionable state of things, would be remedied, if the Government provided the prisoners with food, without the intervention of bunyas, whose abominable chicanery would thus be avoided. Suggestions.

It appears to me that the Government in the month of May, when grain is cheapest ought to buy in a stock of one year's consumption, of wheat, rice, dâl, ghee, salt, pepper, and tobacco, to be stored in a building sufficient for the purpose. No other article of diet, condiments, or stimulants should on any account be served out. The requisite quantity of wheat should be daily ground and sifted by the prisoners selected for the duty. The provisions should be served out at a fixed hour, under proper inspection.

Any extra articles for the sick, whenever required, should be supplied after due consideration by the Medical Officer.

The weekly distribution of pice for shaving, &c. should be abolished: and in lieu of this, two barbers and a malee kept upon the jail establishment.

The well ought to be outside the jail walls, and a water-course should lead from it to the interior of the quadrangle; within which two reservoirs of masonry should be built to receive the water: the one for drinking water, the other to be employed as a bath, and neither should be above three feet deep: at the other extremities of the reservoirs, the water should be allowed to escape beyond the jail wall, so as always to insure a clear supply. A very simple capstan machinery, worked by some of the prisoners, within the jail walls, would draw the requisite quantity of water, whenever needed. Drinking water, often now a subject of complaint, would be then abundant: and in the larger reservoir every healthy prisoner should be compelled to bathe and wash his garments daily.

A portion of ground should be cultivated by some of the prisoners for the production of vegetable supplies, for the whole, in sufficient abundance.

The prisoners ought certainly to be properly and vigilantly worked. Those of particular trades should be encouraged to follow them in prison: and any articles formed should be disposed of, and a portion of the proceeds set apart, to be paid to the prisoner on his release.

DISEASES.

No endemic diseases have fallen under my observation.

Fevers. Of the epidemic diseases fever is the most common, and deserving of notice. Throughout the whole district it may certainly be generally considered a mild and tractable complaint; and, in comparison with other provinces, the proportion of fever among the inhabitants is very small.

During the hottest months and the early part of the rains, the few fevers that prevail are more or less of a continued type: in the height of the rains, the type becomes remittent; and from September to the end of November the type becomes intermittent; and from the end of November to April hardly a case of fever occurs. The number of cases of the first type are very few, of the second rather more, and of the third by far the greatest.

In general the fevers of this district require a considerable degree of depletion to be employed at first, especially in the cases of the young and robust: the degree of depletion being far greatest in the continued, moderate in the remittent, and slight in the intermittent fevers.

In my own practice I found all the fevers tractable: and have not had one fatal case of simple fever, during three years.

Any enlargement on the treatment would seem quite unnecessary, I shall therefore merely say, that after premising the requisite depletion, the proper administration of sulphate of quinine or cinchona bark powder will almost infallibly prevent a return.

Amongst the poorer natives, their own simple employment of bitter tonics, with laxatives and abstinence, effect a more tardy cure. Many also necessarily undergo no treatment, allowing the fever to wear itself out.

The mildness of the fevers is especially proven by the rarity of visceral disorganization amongst those who have been even frequently attacked.

Small-pox often becomes epidemic in the district, and is exceedingly severe and fatal, especially at Ajmeer. It generally appears about the beginning of the hot weather, is most severe when the weather is hottest, and declines as the rains advance. Every fourth or fifth year the disease breaks out more severely, becoming a dreadful scourge, so much so as to be a great check on the increase of the population. Small Pox.

The natives of the city of Ajmeer are very prejudiced regarding vaccination; and when small-pox is not actually virulent, are very apathetic about any prophylactic.

I constantly exerted every effort to introduce and keep up the vaccine disease. This was at all times very difficult, the true disease invariably, even in the best seasons, wearing itself out in a very short time, so that proper vesicles were no longer formed, constantly requiring a new supply from a distant source: and when small-pox was greatly prevalent, and terror would have led many to come forward with their children, I found it impossible (probably on account of the variolous state of the atmosphere) to introduce the proper disease at all. Vaccination

When I happened to have good virus, I always found the greatest difficulty in obtaining a few subjects, by petty bribes, and generally of the lowest and filthiest castes: afterwards most of the parents would spoil the vesicles by rubbing, or applying the juice of palma christi leaves, or tobacco ashes.

The native vaccinator was by no means to be relied on, always appearing to think that he deserved great praise for bringing a few children only about once a month. At the same time I had reason to believe that this man frequently inoculated with variolous matter in the town; such having been his former occupation.

I mention these circumstances to shew what great difficulty appeared on all sides to prevent the effectual introduction of vaccination.

So long as only a few low caste children can be obtained by bribes to their parents, and the most wearisome inculcation to the native vaccinator, the cow-pox will never be able to exert any great influence on the spread of small-pox.

Last season, in Ajmeer alone, nineteen hundred children died of this scourge. The ravages of the disease are visible in almost every face met with; and the number of wholly blind or one-eyed people from this cause is very great.

As it is not only a humane but a profitable object, for Government to endeavour to subdue the small-pox by the introduction of an effectual check on its devastating power, proper measures ought to be pursued. The present system is nearly quite useless.

Suggestion. Ineffectual vaccination, especially owing to the carelessness of native vaccinators, has occasioned great prejudice against it in the minds of many. Let any one compare the scar from the vaccination on the arm of a person vaccinated in England (about the year 1808), with the scars left by the general run of vaccinations in India at the present period, and the greatest difference will be observable. On the arms of many of the children said to have been vaccinated in India, the scar is very faintly perceptible.

The greatest attention ought therefore to be paid to the nature of the virus employed, and to the progress of the vesicle throughout.

I am still confident that the proper vaccine disease will certainly modify in *all* cases; and in *almost all* certainly prevent an attack of small-pox.

To ensure the spread of vaccination more support ought to be given by government: the office must be rendered more respectable, and the time of those employed exclusively devoted to the duty. To trust to native agents will not do; and the European officer, unless rendered of importance in the eyes of the natives, and openly supported by the authorities, will never succeed in disseminating vaccination.

The civil or military medical officer may perhaps vaccinate the whole children of the head town and neighbouring villages of a district; but all these will be very few compared to the number in the whole pergunah.

To send out native vaccinators to the district is quite useless, as their reports cannot be relied upon.

An effectual method of propagating vaccination would seem to be the appointment of superintendents, on remunerating salaries, solely for this duty, in each large province. The superintendent ought to be allowed the requisite number of native assistants, and in every proper way rendered respectable in the eyes of the natives: during the proper season his duties should be itinerary, in the province to which he might be appointed. In this way the superintendent, proceeding from town to town, should remain at each long enough to vaccinate every child who had not had small-pox in the neighbourhood, and subsequently to observe the proper maturation of the vesicles. Thus, the whole children of a pergunah being properly vaccinated in one season, small-pox would almost disappear, and the province in time become free of danger from this source.

The plan I have proposed would, I believe, be an effectual one; but, if the Government will not adopt any such measure, then the present system of vaccination in Upper India had better be discontinued as useless: and inoculation for small-pox encouraged.

The land scurvy has appeared as a severe epidemic in Scorbutus. this district, though I have only met with a few sporadic cases. The disease was found very intractable, yielding slowly to time, medicine and nutritious diet, with the use of vegetable acids, especially the fruit of the anola or aula (Phyllanthus emblica) which is very sour, and also highly astringent: in general, an early change of climate was found necessary.

When the disease appeared, bad grain was considered as the cause; but facts do not seem to warrant this opinion.

The disease subsided as the seasons became milder. Dr. Macnab has given an excellent account of the disorder.

In those cases of scurvy which came under my own observation, I found sulphate of quinine with mineral acids as a tonic, and nourishing vegetable diet, with wine, and the "aula," given plain or as a pickle, an effectual cure. In one bad case, I successfully kept the patient on a diet of raisins with lime-juice, and some sago with wine, and other treatment as before stated, and a gargle of alum in solution, with tincture of myrrh.

Anola Fruit.

I do not myself attribute any peculiar virtue to the anola fruit, which is very commonly used as a pickle, &c. by the natives, and does not seem superior to any other acid vegetable astringent. The anola, however, appears to contain a quantity of gallic acid.

Sporadic Diseases.

Few of the common sporadic diseases require notice. The dracunculus, gordius medinensis or guineaworm is very commonly met with in this district; cases of it are extensively scattered over the west of India; but in no place it is more frequent than in Marwar. From the presence of this worm considerable irritation and inflammation often result; but seldom to a dangerous degree, except from mal-treatment. I have not been able, in this district, to extract the worm at one operation, ás some inflammation is generally present. Perfect rest, with leeching, fomentations, and poultices, gradually rolling up the worm as it yields, will soon effect a cure, by removal of the cause. In some cases the worm dies within its nidus, giving rise to much inflammation and suppuration: the pain is also very great. The same treatment carried to a greater extent, with the use of opiates, and the evacuation of the abscesses formed, will lead to a favourable result.

Gordius Medinensis.

Rheumatismus.

Acute and chronic rheumatism are frequent, especially in the cold season and rains; when catarrhs and other pulmonary complaints are also common.

On the treatment or variety of the other diseases, occasionally met with, any remarks would seem to be here unnecessary.

Opthalmia.

Op thalmia is very severe and common, and probably much dependent on the hard particles of dust impinging on the eyes, during the frequent high winds. I have not met with it, or heard of it, as contagious, or simply epidemic in this district. One variety indeed sometimes occurs, arising from gonorrhœal discharge, being communicated by the fingers to the eyes. This is rare; but, as elsewhere becomes very severe, and is contagious. Ophthalmia, except the last mentioned variety, is very amenable to proper treatment. The natives themselves do not understand the cure of this complaint: they sometimes however succeed in discussing the disease at first; but, much more frequently aggravate it into a severe lingering complaint.

Hereditary Diseases

Podagra. I have heard of gout appearing among some of the Rajpoots, who drink hard; but I never met with any such cases.

Epilepsy. Epilepsy is rarely met with, and is, where seen, hereditary: and in all the instances that came under my notice, malformation of the head was present.

Hepatits. Hepatitis is sometimes met with, and requires vigorous depletory measures.

Dysenteria Dysentery and diarrhœa are rather often met with, during the rains and cold weather: they are easily subdued, when occurring in subjects of any stamina.

Cholera. Common bilious cholera is not unfrequent during the hot season, when melons and cucumbers are abundantly consumed, and is generally easily cured.

Spasmodic cholera appears about once in every seven or eight years, in this district; which is thus for a long period happily exempted, while the neighbouring countries of Kotah, Boonda and Meywar, are almost annually liable to its severest visitations.

When it does break out in the district the severity and duration are fortunately not very great. At first, some deaths occur; but I found the disease generally yield to bleeding and diffusible stimuli, at the beginning; and calomel with tartar emetic, so soon as re-action commenced; followed by purgatives: all the remedia adjuvantia were also employed.

Epizooties Murrians among the cattle sometimes happen. During the height of the Pali plague, at the places infected, cattle, sheep and dogs suffered and died in numbers, from fever, and enlarged glands in the throat and neck. In some animals, observed by me at the time, the swelling of the submaxillary glands was the only affection. Similar diseases of animals are often observed in the Levant and other places during plagues. In the same way, during severe cholera, domestic fowls often die very suddenly in great numbers and apparently of that disease: (at Hoshungabad I frequently observed fowls during severe cholera, turn giddy, pass watery stools and speedily to die.)

Diseases of Plants.

Diseases of plants no doubt exist in this district; but certainly rarely, and never in a very eminent degree. During the presence of scurvy, that disease was at first attributed to the use of bad grain, and a large quantity was destroyed at the time, though the grain presented no peculiar marks of disease, having been merely of an inferior quality; it would therefore seem a pity that such should have been destroyed, especially as the general opinion now is, that the use of the grain was not an exciting cause.

The very innutritious kinds of grain, often used by the poor, sometimes give rise to cutaneous complaints from poverty of blood.

It appears that wheat and barley are never in this district affected by diseases injurious to man; but this exemption does not extend to the southward and westward.

Popular Medicine.

Under this head may be mentioned the common employment of occasional simple laxatives, and by some (generally Mahommedans) periodical bleedings. A vast variety of ridiculous charms are also in use. The treatment of sick animals by the natives is often successful.

Animals, intended for the food of man, are periodically given a considerable quantity of salt and soda (khari nimmuk): and before killing them, are given a large dose by the butchers, to render the flesh soft: the salt does not usually purge the sheep but has the effect of fattening them.

Hospitals.

The small stone-shed, used as a jail hospital, has been already alluded to: the only other is the magazine hospital, appropriated particularly to the magazine, but also used for the general reception of cases.

This hospital is situated nearly opposite to the main entrance of the magazine, on the opposite side of the public road, in the centre of a piece of ground about eighty yards square, not protected from the road by any wall or screen.

The hospital is a stone vaulted building, containing one central ward, thirty feet long by twenty broad; and has the usual verandah space around, divided by the corners into four compartments, in the outer wall of each of which there is on unglazed door.

There is a small room in one verandah for the reception of medicines, &c.

Rats burrow through the pukka floor of the hospital, and the medicines, &c. can never be properly preserved, so long as this is the case: the nature of the shelves put up is not efficient to protect the phials, &c. placed upon them: these defects might be easily remedied.

The two small windows in the surgery, and two of the doors, should be glazed and well fitted to their frames.

The space around the hospital should be inclosed by a low wall, to prevent the passage across of carts, cattle or noisy people, now a frequent nuisance.

This hospital is sufficient in size for the healthy climate of Ajmeer: and is in a well drained airy situation.

On my first arrival at Ajmeer I proposed the establishment of an hospital for the poor, which I, of course, volunteered to superintend; but the proposal was not encouraged.

Medical Duties.

Notwithstanding the salubrity of the climate, the medical duties are sometimes severe; owing to the great distance apart of the officers' houses, and the number of European writers, and warrant officers with their families; the total under the medical charge is upwards of eight hundred.

While at Ajmeer the medical officer performs all the agency, civil, magazine and guard medical duties. When the Agent to the Governor General marches, the medical officer usually accompanies him, and the Ajmeer charge is made over temporarily to some other medical officer, who receives one hundred rupees per mensem, on the agreement of visiting Ajmeer at least once a week.

Spontaneos Cures.

As Dr. Hennen remarked, the generality of diseases have not a natural tendency to terminate in death; and this is fully exemplified at Ajmeer, where by far the greatest number of cases, among the poorer natives, recover spontaneously.

Practice of Physic and Surgery. The practice of medicine among the natives, is in the hands of Mahommedan hakims, and Hindoo bueds, naies, baburs, and jetties. Their knowledge appears to be at a very low ebb; their chief reliance is upon charms and signs; the materials of their prescriptions, often the most incongruous and laughable even to themselves, when they are asked on what principles they prescribe, and the methods of action of the various substances.

Their practice, I believe, is generally innocent; with exception of that of the "jetties," who are superstitiously respected by all of the Jain faith, and as no inquiries would be made by natives, they have great facilities for doing harm.

In simple external complaints, with the exception of eye diseases, the common practice may be beneficial; but, it appears evident, from the usual inefficiency of the practice, that those who escape are carried through only by strength of constitution.

The state of surgery is sufficiently good, in the treatment of incised wounds: union by the first intention being almost always effected, the native constitution also greatly aiding in this: the edges of the wound are generally brought accurately together, and the dried skin of the "sambur" is ground very fine with water, and applied in a paste over the edges: this speedily dries and keeps the parts in close contact: the gelatinous nature of the application also probably tends to promote immediate union.

Operations for cataract are successfully performed, at times, by travelling oculists, whose employment is hereditary: they know nothing of anatomy whatever; and operate quite fearlessly.

Of the greater operations of surgery, lithotomy is sometimes performed: the lithotomist is as ignorant as the oculist in regard to anatomy; yet, he operates quite fearlessly, generally with bungling violence; and sometimes succeeds.

If the European surgeon, with his science, only possessed the self-sufficiency and indifference of these native operators, his success would be insured.

In regard to the materia medica, many productions now imported from other places, may be found indigenous; but the indolence of the inhabitants, and their propensity to opium, and other intoxicating drugs, has almost entirely prevented them making any researches on such subjects. Materia Medica.

Almost without exception, the wealthy inhabitants of Ajmeer, from early dissipation, become impotent or in a state tending that way, though in full manhood as to years; and as such people will pay well for relief, a great number of substances are employed in the most preposterous manner with the view of benefitting in that way; hence a great part of the Ajmeer pharmacopœia consists of substances employed from their supposed aphrodisiac virtues.

Nearly all the articles of real efficacy, used by the natives, are found in our own pharmacopœia, such as gamboge, impure calomel, pure corrosive sublimate, arsenious acid, senna, cassia fistula, sulphur, mercury, opium, musk, castor, croton tiglium, rhubarb, turbeth root, jalap (from Mirabilis jalapæ), impure potash, soda, the impure mineral acids, &c. &c. &c.

On making inquiry, regarding the greatest number of articles, the reply of the hakims and punsaris is, that the efficacy is not in the substance itself, but in the combination: and that a person may take a chittack of it without injury.

I shall now subjoin a list of a number of articles selected by the punsaris and myself from the nominal three thousand thailies (or bags), that are kept in their shops: the three hundred arranged by me, are all those to which the punsaris themselves attach any importance.

Asgandh, असगंध : Isgandh, इसगंध : Ashwagandah, अश्वगंधा : Physalis flexuosa. This plant is commonly found all over India; the roots are employed medicinally, and are considered good in rheumatic and dyspeptic disorders, especially those accompanied by flatulency: they are of a warm nature, calculated to promote all the secretions. The root is not given alone; but is combined with other medicines and mesalihs.

Alusa, अलुसा : Arus, अरुस : Bakas, बाकस : Justicia Adhatoda. Common all over India. Leaves are chiefly used at Ajmeer, and are considered diaphoretic and sedative, and used in cough prescriptions. The root is used in Ceylon as an emmenagogue, and to cause abortion. The charcoal of the plant is used to make gunpowder.

Asaloo, असालु. A small plant cultivated about Ajmeer: the seeds are used and are heating, promote the secretions: they are also taken in milk to strengthen the body: much used in mesalihs of camels: to the taste are bitter and hot.

Ajwayan, अजवायन : Ligusticum Ajowan. Is a species of lovage, cultivated about Ajmeer (and all over India): the seeds are highly carminative; promote the secretions: good in dyspepsia: much used in all mesalihs: eight seers for one rupee.

Ajmod, अजमोद : Ajmot, अजमोठ : Apium involucratum. Is a species of smallage: very hot and carminative: good in dyspepsia: much used in all mesalihs: is brought to Ajmeer from Harowtee and Mewar: four seers for one rupee.

Apheem, अफीम : Opium. Papaver Somniferum. Used to great excess as a stimulant, by almost all classes: also given in medicine as a sedative, and to check diarrhœa; the price varies according to the quality. The poppy is much cultivated in Rajpootanah.

Khorasani Ajmot, षोरासानी अजमोट : a species of Apium. The seed is brought from Persia: is very hot and carminative.

Khorasani Ajwayan, षोरासानी अजवायन : Hyosciamus niger. The seed is sold and comes from Persia: is used as a stimulant: also in the mesalihs of animals.

Amultas ka phul, अमलतासकाफल : Kirmala ka phul, कीरमालाकाफल : Cassia fistula. The pods are brought to Ajmeer from Mewar (the tree however grows at Ramghur in the district); the internal black pulp, attached to the sepimenta, is used as a laxative, taken diffused in water; or, four or five tolas are taken with senna leaves. One seer of the fruit yields twenty tolas of the concrete pulp, which is sold at four seers for one rupee. The bark of the root of this tree I have found to act as a very strong purge.

Anola, अनोला : Aola, औला : Phyllanthus emblica: Emblic Myrobalan. The tree is cultivated at Ajmeer; the fruit is brought from Kotah and Mewar: it is used abundantly fresh or dried as a condiment, being pickled also; and in dying, and to wash the hair with: the fruit is very acid and astringent, and contains gallic acid. The use of this fruit was supposed beneficial as an adjuvant in treating the scurvy at Nusseerabad.

Aritha, अरीथा : Ritha, रीथा : Sapindus saponaria : Soap-nut. The dried berries are brought from Kotah, Malwa, and Mewar; they are not used in medicine; but, are much employed in dying, and as a detergent: eight seers are sold for the rupee.

Achu, आचु : Al, आल : Morinda multiflora, and tinctoria. Small species of Morinda, cultivated throughout Rajpootanah, principally near Kotah, and all over Harowtee. The plant is allowed to remain three years in the ground, and then the roots are taken up and dried. The dye is a fine turkey red, and is very plentiful. One maund costs sixteen rupees. Is not used medicinally.

Anardana, अनारदाना : Naspal, नासपाल : Punica granatum : Pomegranate. The dried seeds with their fleshy envelopes are sold, and used in sherbets: are plentiful at Ajmeer, considered cooling. Naspal is the bark of the fruit, and is only used in dying. The bark of the root though strongly purgative is not used in medicine. Large quantities of fine pomegranates are annually brought from Cabul to Ajmeer.

Abhrak, अभ्रक : Mica or Talc. Very abundant about Ajmeer: different sorts by exposure to heat assume a variety of colours: sold in powder for medical purposes, and is taken in the dose of one tola to strengthen the body.

Akakiya, अकाकीया. A red stone brought from Delhie, containing iron: is used as a tonic, in the dose of one tola: one seer for two rupees,

Aptimun, आपतीमुन : Amr-bel, अमरबेल. Is the yellow colored parasite so often seen on babul trees, all over India, and very common at Ajmeer. The entire plant is used in medicine: it is a creeper: is given in "munjus," which is a diluent form of medicine, employed preparatory to giving a purge.

Aptimun wilayti: Extract of the plant from Bombay: used in the same way: one tola for eight annas.

Akut, अकुट : Chooni, चुनी : small rubies or garnets. Are brought viâ Pali: are used as an aphrodisiac: one tola for two rupees.

Anisun, आनीसुन : Pimpinella Anisum : Aniseed. Imported viâ Pali: considered carminative: also much used in rheumatism: one seer for three rupees eight annas.

Aprang, आपरंग : Rangbharat, रंगभरत : Damlakwaypi, दमलकवेपा : Hira-dukhan, हीरादखन : A gum resin. A beautiful kind of kino, brought from Bombay : considered very astringent : is given in intestinal hœmorrhages : is also used in enamelling on gold : four tolahs for one rupee.

Abresham, आबरेशम. White slik, cut unto very minute pieces ; is used to remedy impotence : four tolas for one rupee.

Ak, आक : Mudar, मदार : Asclepias gigantea. Is very plentiful ; but, is not kept as a drug by either "punsaris" or "attars." The natives of Ajmeer, only use the milk of the plant, and the leaves, which they apply for rheumatism. I have found the bark of the root, given in continued and large doses, very effectual in healing leprous and other indolent ulcers, and in all cutaneous diseases, accompanied by a want of action. This medicine acts strongly on the skin, increasing perspiration, and occasioning a general sense of formication. The powdered bark is also an excellent emetic, generally effectual in the dose of one scruple, and I have, for years, used it as such, amongst the poor classes.

Amber, आमबर. A mixed sort of scent, of the consistence of a plaster, made up by "attars :" is heating : chiefly used as aphrodisiac : seems an imitation of ambergris. One tolah costs five rupees six annas. Natives of Ajmeer do not know real amber.

Bhai-birrung, भैबीरंग. Seed of a plant brought from Harowtee : are considered warm : used in mesalihs, and in prescriptions to promote digestion.

Bhai-phamba, भैफमबा. Flowers of a plant brought from Harowtee : considered warm : used to promote digestion.

Bharangi, भारंगी : Verbesina prostrata. The bark of the stem of the small plant is brought from Harowtee : considered warm : used to promote digestion.

Bid-ari-khand, बीदारीखंद. Root of a climber found in the Ajmeer hills : considered of a warm nature : used among the great number of ingredients of many prescriptions.

Bijban, बीजबान. Seed of a plant found in all Rajpootanah : is heating : used in aphrodisiac prescriptions.

Bunafsha, बनाफशा : Viola odorifera : Sweet violet. The whole plant is brought dried from Delhie : is considered of a warm nature : is prescribed in fevers.

Bartung, बारतंग. Seed of a bush : is brought from Delhie : considered cooling, and astringent : used in sherbets, in diarrhœa.

Badam, बादाम : Almonds. Very much used at Ajmeer, as restoratives; come from Cabul viâ Beekaneer. One maund costs twenty rupees.

Bho-phulli, भोफली: A small scandent plant, abundant about Ajmeer: contains a great quantity of mucus: is used, rubbed up with water and strained, in great quantity, as an aphrodisiac: is also considered cooling, and used in prescriptions as such.

Barjuri, बेरजुरी. Bark of the root of a climber found in Rajwarra: is tasteless: one fourth of a tola is a dose: is given to women after child-birth, in "luddoo:" said to augment the secretion of milk: to relieve the after-pains, and to strengthen.

Bhilawa, भीलावा : Bhilawan : Semicarpus anacardium. Is the nut of a large forest tree of the same name, common in Delhie and Harowtee, the acrid viscid oil the nut contains is used as an escharotic, as a counter-irritant: it leaves a mark for life: it creates great pain and often very bad sores; but, ignorant natives, unacquainted with our blisters, have a greater dread of them than of the Bhilawa: is given in medicine in small doses, and is considered a stimulant and narcotic: is much used in the mesalihs of elephants; given in large doses, it renders these animals furious: is considered good in venereal diseases, especially of women: the farina of the anthers of the flowers is very narcotic and irritating: people of a peculiar habit accidentally sleeping under the tree when in blossom, or even going near the flowers, are stupified and have their faces and limbs swollen: the mature corolla and the receptacle are fleshy and sweetish sour, and are eaten roasted or boiled as a vegetable, and aphrodisiac along with cocoanut and chironjies. It is thus used in a prescription for the venereal disease of women: the mercury, henbane and bhilawa being the active ingredients.

Quicksilver,	4 massee.
Khorasani ajwayan,	6 ditto.
Ajmot,	6 ditto.
Ajwayan,	5 ditto.
Ukulkurra,	4 ditto.
Bhilawa,	2 nuts.
Gour	½ a chittack.

Pounded, mixed and made into balls as big as a wild "byer:" one a day for a dose: the patient is said to recover in seven days.

Maloni Bapchi, मालोनी बापची. Seed of a small plant found about

Ajmeer ; tasteless ; has a fine scent : is of a warm nature : a dram is given in medicine : used externally with other medicines to cure the itch.

Bapchi, बापची. Seed of a small bush found near Ajmeer ; is very mucilaginous, cooling and demulcent : is taken in sherbet.

Bahira, बाहीरा : Terminalia bellerica : Belleric Myrobalan. Fruit of the tree, brought from Malwa, Kotah and other places : very astringent : considered cooling, and given in hematuria : much used in dying, and in mesalihs : common in all bazars : eight seers for one rupee.

Baboona-soorookh, बाबुनासुरख : Anthemis nobilis. Camomile The root is imported viâ Bombay : is taken as an aphrodisiac, and general tonic : one rupee a seer.

Baboona-sufaid, बाबुनासफैद. White root of a similar nature, from the same place : used as an aphrodisiac.

Be-dana, बेदाना. Said to be the seeds of the quince (Pyrus tomentosa) ; but they appear more like dried mulberry seeds (Morus nigra) : the tree in Cabul is called " bai : " are demulcent and cooling : very mucilaginous : are used in sherbets : one seer costs four rupees.

Bans-lochan, बंसलोचन : Tabashir, ताबाशीर. A silicious concrete of a pure white colour, and brittle consistency, found in the hollow joints of the bamboo. I have often removed it from old bamboos at Hoshungabad. This comes to Ajmeer from Hurdwar : is used as aphrodisiac ; and in general debility. One massa is the dose : two tolaa for one rupee. N. B. Like most other native medicines, is quite inert, of course.

Bal-chur, बालछर : (Valeriana Jatamansi : Spikenard ?) Found near standing water at Ajmeer : the roots are small and knotty, and fine like hair, hence the name : have a sweet scent : are tasteless : used to heat, strengthen and excite the system : one tola is the dose ; are very much used also in hair mesalihs : two seers for one rupee. Also the name of a grass, the roots of which are like fine hair, sweet-scented, and much used in cleaning the hair. This latter grass is the Andropogon schænanthus.

Bel, बेल : Belgar, बेलगार : Ægle marmelos : Cratæva marmelos : Bengal quince. The tree is found in the Ajmeer hills, and is abundant in Kotah : the fruit is chiefly used : the ripe pulp is spongy and nearly tasteless, and the seeds are surrounded by a strong clear gum ; this gum is useful to cement fine paper articles

Here the natives consider the fruit cooling, wholesome and somewhat astringent: used medicinally in diarrhœa: the pericarp is very hard, brittle, and has a delicious smell, on which account an "atr" is extracted from it in the Dukhan. The leaves are sacred to Matajee (from the milk of whose breast this tree is believed to have sprung up). The punsaris believe that one pice's size of the bark of the root of this tree, rubbed up with ghee, will, if given soon, recover a person who has taken an overdose of opium.

Bhidaira, भीदैरा. Root of a small bush found in Ajmeer, and brought also from Delhie: has little taste: used in medicine: women take it during pregnancy, believing it to cause the womb to rise out of the pelvis when tardy in so doing.

Bol ka gond, बोलकागोंद: Bija bol, बीजाबोल. A dark reddish yellow opaque gum resin, like myrrh (appears to be true myrrh) imported via Bombay. The natives have a curious idea regarding this gum, that by eating it or even rubbing it in the teeth, they will become loose and fall out: it is considered a warm medicine: is given to children in enlarged abdomen, mixed with musabbur (aloes) as a deobstruent: is also used in making native ink: one seer costs eleven annas.

Beg-bunupsa, बेगबनपशा. Iris Florentina. Orris Root. Root of a small plant brought from Delhie: used as a fine scent in medicine; and in compounding "atrs."

Bisfay aj, बीसफेयाज: Bisfaij, बीसफैज: Polypodium vulgare: Common Fern. The root is brought from Arabia via Bombay; considered heating, and given in flatulence, and indigestion: not considered poisonous in any quantity: one seer costs four rupees.

Bikhma, बीषमा: apparently a tuberous root of a species of Aconite (Aconitum atees, or heterophyllum). The root is small, clean, soft to the knife, of a very strong pleasant bitter taste: one or two massee are given ground up in ghee, and the dose is said to cure colic pains speedily.: is much used in medicine: is poisonous in a large quantity: one tola costs eight annas.

Bhirmi-sugan, भीरमीसुगान. Leaves of a small plant brought from Delhie, employed in making scents.

Bhirmi-vidaya, भीरमीवीदेया. Leaves of a climber from Mount Aboo: are very stimulating: used in the "seet" disease, a sort of catalepsy.

Barug-sudab, बारगसुदाब. Leaves of a plant from Delhie: are heating and as such used in medicine to cure flatulency and dyspepsia; two rupees for one seer.

Bura-armani, बडाआरमानी ; Yellow Armenian Bole : Gila-armani : गीलाआरमानी : Red Armenian Bole. Both used in the same way, as astringent and cooling : one tola or six massee are taken as a dose in diarrhœa : they are brought from Delhie : one seer costs two rupees.

Bojidan, बोजीदान. Root of a small plant from Delhie : heating, and used to strengthen, and as an aphrodisiac ; one seer costs two rupees.

Bekh-kurpus, बेखकरपस. Root of a small plant, comes from Delhie : heating ; one seer costs two rupees.

Bekh-unjubaz, बेखअनजुबाज. Red-coloured root of a plant, that is brought from Delhie ; considered as cooling and astringent.

Budranja-boya, बदरंजाबोया. A species of melissa, a small plant found about Ajmeer, considered heating, used to cleanse the blood : one seer for two rupees.

Babai, बाबैय : Ocymum pilosum ; Ciliated Basil. Very common in all the khets ; the leaves have a very fragrant smell, exactly like verbena : the plant is used to prevent the approach of insects, especially of bugs ; the seeds are mucilaginous.

Chireta, चीरैता : Kirayta, कीरैता : Gentiana Chereytta. The whole dry plant is brought from Pali and Delhie : much used in decoction as tonic and febrifuge : one maund costs ten rupees.

Cabab-chiny, काबाबचीनी : Seetul-chiny, शीतलचीनी : Piper cubeba ; Cubebs. Cubebs are brought via Pali : considered cooling : used in mesalihs given to promote digestion : are esteemed an excellent condiment : not used to cure gonorrhœa : one seer for twelve annas.

Chitruk, चीटरक : Chitraka, Lal Chitruk ; Plumbago Zeylanica. A small plant found near Ajmeer ; the root is considered heating : used internally to promote digestion : is also epispastic and rubifacient : used as a sialagogue.

Chuka ka bij, चुकाकाबीज : Rumex acetosa ; Sorrel. The seed is considered cooling and astringent ; is cultivated.

Chhuwara, Chhuhara, छुहारा : Phœnix dactylifera. Dates are brought from Bombay viâ Pali ; are very much eaten : are considered restorative : one maund costs ten rupees.

Chunigond, चुनीगोंद : Palas pipal ka gond, पलासपीपलकागोंद : Dak ka gond, ढाककागोंद : Butea frondosa. The Indian kino : considered very cooling and astringent : very cheap.

Chundun, चनदण : Sandal, समदल ; Santalum album ; Sirium myrtifolium : White and Yellow Sandal Wood or Saunders : Comes viâ Pali : is used in medicine, and considered cooling ; but, is chiefly used in worshipping, and to adorn the bodies of certain castes : one maund costs twenty-six rupees.

Rakht-chundun, रकतचनदन : Lal chundun : Pterocarpus Santalinus : Red Saunders. Is used chiefly in suffumigations to the native gods ; is also used in medicine : is brought from Delhie : costs ten rupees per maund.

Gopi-chundun, गोपीचनदन. An aluminous yellow earth, brought from the Ganges at Hurdwar, used to mark the foreheads of those who worship Vishnu : also given in medicine.

Chokha, चोखा. Root of a plant that is brought from Delhie : is heating : taken internally as narcotic : is bitter : chiefly used mixed with sulphur and oil to cure the itch in camels.

Chob-chini, चोबचीनी : Smilax Chinensis : China root. Comes viâ Bombay : it is a largish, insipid, whitish root, in slices : is taken as restorative and aphrodisiac in milk : one tola is a dose : used also in mesalihs : one seer costs two rupees. N. B. Natives suppose that this is the root of the "hazari," marygold (Tagetes erecta), after being in the ground three years.

Churrus, चरस : Cannabis sativa : Hemp. This is the extract of the hemp plant ; and also the natural resin that exudes on the leaves : the first is very inferior, and is made artificially by evaporating the expressed juice ; the second is collected by natives in leather garments, who early in the morning pass through the wild hemp plants, when a quantity of resinous exudation adheres to the leather, and is afterwards scraped off ; this forms the best churrus, which is used to intoxicate, and as an aphrodisiac drug : one massee smoked, creates inebriety in one unused to it ; one seer costs eight or ten rupees ; the best comes from Nepal.

Charul, चारल : Chironji, चीरोंजी : Buchanania latifolia : Chironjia sapida. The chironji is the seed removed from the small stone of the "achhar" fruit : it is brought to Ajmeer from Kotah : the seed is very palatable and nutritious, especially when roasted : is used also in medicine, and considered heating : one seer and a half cost a rupee. The fresh fruit is very agreeable.

Chumpouti, चमपौडी. Berry of a small plant, brought viâ Pali : used in scents and also in medicine : one seer for one rupee.

Chakowar, चकोवार : Jangli-powar, जंगलीपोवार : Cassia obtusifolia. The seed of the plant is used in medicine : the plant is scarce about Ajmeer, is prescribed to cleanse the blood, in an entire state; when the seeds are pounded and then swallowed, vomiting is produced: the leaves of the young plant are eaten as a vegetable; are also applied in itch cases: (is very common in the Dukhan :) goats and sheep are fond of the seed; one seer of the seed costs one pice.

Chak, Chuk, चुक. An extract: very sour: eaten to give appetite and promote digestion. Probably the extract of "chuka," or sorrel: one tola for one anna.

Chumbranuk, चमबरानक. A single valve of the muscle shell without the fish: used as an aphrodisiac.

Sitanuk, शीटानक. One valve of a muscle shell, with the dried fish attached. The punsaris call it "the small head of a sea animal:" used as an aphrodisiac, and also said to cure the cynanche of children: comes from Bombay viâ Pali: one seer costs two rupees.

Castoori, Kustoori, कसतुरी. This is the name given to musk; which is also called "mushuk:" at Ajmeer the punsaris do not know castor as a distinct substance by this name: good musk is not to be had at Ajmeer.

Chundrus, चंद्रस: Copal resin. Is brought viâ Pali: the fine shavings of it are used in medicine to stop hœmoptysis; made up into a medicine called "khairwa;" is much used in varnishes: one maund costs thirty-five rupees.

Cajuputi ka tel, Ilachie ka tel, इलाचीका तेल: Melalenea leucodendron. Native "attars" sell this oil very pure at Ajmeer; they only know it as oil of cardamoms: it comes from Bombay: is applied by women to refrigerate their eyelids: used as a carminative and rubefacient: one seer costs twenty-four rupees.

Cratæva Tapia: Polyandria Monogynia. Garlick Pear: Hind: Burua. A common tree on the hornblende schist rocks of Ajmeer. In May the tree is in profuse blossom and presents a splendid appearance, the flowers being blue and buff. The foliage is very ornamental, and the wood is used to make necklaces of. This hardy tree would be a great desideratum in "compounds."

Dhuniya, धनीया: Coriandrum sativum: Coriander seed. Is cultivated all over Rajpootanah: as usual used as a condiment; and in mesalihs of animals: the green plant is called "khôtmeer," and is much used, made into "chutnee:" the seed costs four rupees a maund.

Dalchini, दालचीनी: Laurus Cinnamomum : Cinnamon. Is brought from Delhie and Pali : not much used by the natives : does not appear to be good at Ajmeer : one seer for one rupee.

Daru-arad, दारुआरद : Daru-huldi. Large yellow root, of a tree, from Delhie : is tasteless : considered heating and carminative : one pice's size taken is said to cure flatulency and indigestion : it is taken mixed with a nostrnm called " cur-sut."

Datuni, दातुनी : Croton tiglium. This is the root of the " jumalgota" plant : brought from Delhie and Pali : it is a very powerful purge : much used in prescriptions : one seer costs four rupees.

Darun-aj-akarbi, दारुनआजआकरबी. A kind of fern : the root and leaves of which come from Arabia viâ Bombay : considered as a tonic : four to six massee are a dose : one tola costs two rupees.

Dhaura ka phool, धौराकाफुल : Grislea tomentosa. The scarlet flowers come from Kotah and Harowtee generally : are considered stimulating, and given to women in labour : are also used in dying : one seer costs four annas. The gum of this tree, called dhaura or dhan ka gond is brought from Mewar and Harowtee, and is abundant, white in colour, like the katira and tragacanth gums, swells in water ; in dying cloth it is applied to those parts that the dye is not wished to touch : it is eaten in " luddoo :" one maund costs ten rupees.

Dhatura (white), धातुरा : Kanak (black), कनक : Kanak bij (the seed) : Datura fastuosa and metel, &c. The seed only is used by the natives, eaten as a stimulant or given as a narcotic in medicine ; or, with the intention of robbing or murdering the individual who has taken it : in the latter case it is given in sweetmeats. The natives do not smoke the plant : the greatest benefit is however derived from smoking the whole plant in asthma : and as an antispasmodic and anodyne in other affections of the natives.

Dudiya-mura, दुद्दीयामुरा : Vishnag : Bishnag. A small root, similar in appearance to huldi : is brought mixed with the huldi of commerce : is considered poisonous, and is separated by the punsaris : is also distinctly imported : is more yellow than common huldi : one tola is said to prove fatal : is used in medicine.

The following may be considered a good instance of the incongruous ingredients of the native " noshkas" (or prescriptions) : and the application of the remedy an instance of the gross extravagance of the native practice.

Kuchla pounded (nux vomica seed)....	1 tola.
White kanel root (neri um odorum)....	1 ditto.
Dudiya-mara, (aconitum (?))	1 ditto.
Ukul-kurra, (canna indica)	1 ditto.
Kendi ka bij (palma christi)..........	1 ditto.
Lal phitkari (red alum)...............	1 ditto.
Manisil (red sulphuret of arsenic)......	1 ditto.
Pokhur-mo..........................	1 ditto.
Dal-chini (cinnamon).................	1 ditto.
Loban (gum benjamin)	1 ditto.
Kala tel (black mustard oil)..........	4 pice bhur.

These are pounded and put into a quarter of a seer of mustard oil, and let to stand for five or six days, and then distilled: an oil comes over that is a powerful vesicatory: it is used as a rubefacient in rheumatism; but principally as an aphrodisiac. The native hakims apply it to the penis wrapping up the penis in pawn leaves: it remains applied during three days: the second day it blisters: the third day it removes the integuments; during the healing of the sore produced, the itching and irritation cause venereal appetite.

The oil obtained must be in very small quantity as, of course, the mustard oil will not distil:

Dhantari, धंतारी. Seed of a plant brought from Harowtee: is used in compound medicines.

Dus-mula, दसमुला. Said to be the woods of the ten trees brought from Odeypoor; when a woman is purged in labour, by giving this the diarrhœa is supposed to be checked.

Dudi, दुदी. A small plant about Ajmeer: considered cooling: taken in weakness creates blood.

Dal-shikara, Dal-chikara, दालचीकारा. A crystallized salt, brought from Bombay: it is white and transparent, in small grains: it is very poisonous: is sometimes used in medicine; but, chiefly in "rasan" or transmutation of metals: is true perchloride of mercury, or corrosive sublimate: costs one rupee per tola.

N. B. It is as soluble as English corrosive sublimate, and has the same taste and appearance, and yields the same brick-red precipitate with sub-carbonate of potassa.

Dalchini ka tel, दालचीनीकातेल : Oil of Cinnamon. Is brought from Bombay : considered heating : used as a carminative and rubefacient : three tolas for one rupee.

Dana-buti, दानाबुती. A small plant found about Ajmeer, which is dried, and when taken as medicine, considered cooling : applied pounded checks the discharge from ulcers.

Elwa, एलवा : Mus-abbur, मुसाबर : Aloe perfoliata : Extract of Aloe plant. Brought from Bombay : considered heating : used as a purge with myrrh (bol ka gond) : two seers for one rupee.

The leaves of the fresh plant are also applied pounded, to bruises, &c. &c. ; the plant is cultivated in gardens.

Guj-pipar, गजपीपार. Supposed to be the root of Borassus flabelliformis : brought from Cabul : is astringent and is given in medicine, to promote digestion : one seer costs two rupees ; the guj peepul or guj-pipar is the sliced dried fruit of Pothos officinalis.

Gur-batas, गरबातास. Root of a climber brought from Delhie : has a bad smell : is considered astringent and cooling : much used in horse mesalihs : four seers for one rupee.

Gajuba, गाजुबा. Leaves and triangular stalks of a small succulent plant, brought from Bombay ; heating, and used as a purge.

Gokhru, Gokhara, गोखरु : Tribulus terrestris and lanuginosus. Caltrops. The seed is highly mucilaginous : as is the whole plant : is cooling and demulcent, taken in water as a diluent. Very abundant and troublesome to the naked feet of the natives.

Gorakmundi, गोरखमुनदी : Sphœranthus mollis and indica. A small plant common near water banks at Ajmeer : has a round pink blossom : considered heating : cleanses the blood : aphrodisiac : also opens the bowels : the flower and seed capsules are used.

Ganda-birosa (virosa), गंदाबीरोसा : Salaie, Salar : Boswellia thurifera. The tree is very plentiful in the Ajmeer hills : the gunda-birosa is the prepared gum resin of this tree, and is similar in appearance and qualities to Venice turpentine : is brought from Mewar, Harowtee and the Shekhawattee hills : considered stimulating : an oil is distilled from it, said to cure gonorrhœa : used also in ointments : much used in painting, and by the lakheries : one maund costs twelve rupees.

Gugal ka gond, गुगलकागोंद : Amyris agallocha. The tree is plentiful in the Ajmeer hills : yields a fragrant gum resin : used in the sacred fumigations by the brahmuns : the gum has a similarity to myrrh : used also in flatulencies taken in ghee : is one of the ingredients in the incense or "dhoop."

Gari-gond, गारीगोंद. A light substance like the decayed cotyledons of a seed, or decayed soft grains of the pith of wood : is very bitter to the taste. The punsaris call it a foreign white gum : it is a purge, and given when vision is much obstructed from any cause : one massee with other ingredients is a dose.

Gul-gajuba, गुलगाजुबा. Flowers of gajuba from Bombay : cooling, in various mixed prescriptions : one seer costs two and a half rupees.

Gao-lochan, गावलोचन. Gall stones, extracted from the gall bladders of dead cows : much used in medicine : also in charms ; and in painting.

Gandhak ka araq, गंधककाअरक. Weak impure sulphuric acid, brought from Bombay : sold by "attars :" reckoned corroborant, cooling, and to increase the appetite : sixteen drops are taken in water : one tola costs one rupee.

Gandhak, गंधक : Sulphur. There are three varieties : brought from Bombay viâ Pali, Shekhawattee and Delhie. Ourasar gundhuk is very pure, crystallized in green masses, semi-transparent ; and is the dearest and least used ; costs three rupees for one seer. Antiya gundhuk, yellow sulphur, extracted near Surat, commonest sort, and most used in gunpowder ; one seer costs about six annas. Nirmulasar gundhuk, comes from Pali and Bombay, is of a yellowish white colour, used in medicine to cure the itch : one seer costs one rupee.

Habubir, हाबुबीर. A small fruit from Delhie ; is cooling : has a slight smell and is used by attars : two seers for one rupee.

Haribir, हारीबीर. A fruit brought dried from Harowtee : is bitterish and astringent : used in medicine.

Haldi, हलदी : Curcuma longa : Turmeric. Is brought from Mewar and Harowtee : costs eight rupees a maund.

Hing, हींग : Ferula Asafœtida : Asafœtida. Is brought from Bhahawulpoor in Sind, and from Beekaneer : much used in mesalihs, and eaten by Mohammedans. The white sort costs one rupee a seer, and the red sort three rupees a seer.

Har, हार : Harra, हाड़ा : Terminalia chebula, and other varieties, three in number (beng all the discarded myrobalans of our old pharmacopœias). The myrobalan are brought from Delhie and Harowtee, Hindusthan and the Dukhan : are of four kinds ; namely :

Gural harra, astringent and purgative: used in mesalihs: given in medicine to children: four seers for one rupee.

Juwal harra, used in medicine as a laxative and tonic, and eaten to give an appetite and promote digestion: two seers for one rupee.

Jangi harra, used in the same way: eight seers for one rupee.

Chaipal harra, used only in dying: ten seers for one rupee.

The whole are much used in dying. According to the size of the myrobalan, its value augments; so that a very large one may be worth one hundred rupees or more; the natives believing that the very large ones have the virtue of causing purging by being merely retained in the hands.

Hans-raj, हंसराज: Paraisoo-oosa. Leaves of a common plant found near water at Ajmeer: are heating and febrifuge.

Hurtal, हरताल: Persulphuret of Arsenic: Orpiment. There are two kinds, viz.

Gobheri hurtal, in yellow flakes, used in oil painting: one seer costs one rupee four annas.

Tabki hurtal, greenish, crystallized: given by fakeers in fumigation: one ruttee of it is wrapped up in a leaf of "muggar-bel," and smoked in a hookah: it is evident that the smoker only escapes dangerous consequences, owing to the heat volatilizing most of the arsenic; as it is, the little inhaled often makes the person senseless; salt is then given to restore the senses: thus employed, tabki hurtal is considered a most powerful aphrodisiac: it is also used in ointments: costs three rupees for one seer.

Hira-kussees, हीराकसीस: Dry Persulphate of Iron. Is brought viâ Pali: used in dying and in making ink, blacking leather, &c.: is only used in medicine, made up into "missi" to apply to the teeth, viz.:

Black missi.—Hira-kussees, chaipal harra, chooni gond, lila tootiya, iron filings, kuth, equal parts, pounded and mixed, rubbed on the gums.

White missi.—Sufaid soorma (crystallized carbonate of lime, double refracting spar), and cinnamon pounded together: used as tooth-powder.

Sada-kussees, साढ़ाकसीस. Impure sulphate of Iron, the refuse from the manufactory of the sulphate of copper: four seers for one rupee.

Hazrut-zahoor, हजरतजाहूर : Hazrut-bo, हजरतबो : Aluminite (carbonate of alumina) (?) : A whitish blue hard stone in concretions, like the seed of a date, brought from Cabul : is soft and easily scraped into powder : adheres to the tongue : is insoluble in water : dissolves with effervescence in diluted nitric acid, from which it is precipitated in flocculi by ammonia. The punsaris think this the seed of a fruit, whose stony appearance was caused by the curse of a fakeer : it is considered very cooling, and that two massee taken in water, will create a flow of urine : one tola costs eight annas. This, like most of the native medicines, is quite inert.

Ilachi-dana, इलाचीदाना : Elettaria Cardamomun, (Chhota ilachi, the smallest.)

Amomum Cardamomum, (middle sized.)

Amomum Grana Paradisi, (the largest.)

Cardamom seed is brought from Guzerat, viâ Pali, and from the Dukhan by Kotah : the seeds are universally used in pawn and mesalihs; and in medicine as carminatives. The smallest sort are by far the best, and cost from five to eight rupees a seer. The largest sort are sold at two seers for one rupee, and are much used in mesalihs.

Isabgol, इसबगोल : Ispagul, इसपागुल : Plantago Ispagula :
The seeds of this small plant are used in medicine as mucilaginous : it is cultivated, and sometimes used as food by the poor. The seeds, as astringent, are given in diarrhœa.

Isband, इसबंद : Ermul. Seed of a plant from Marwar ; also found about Ajmeer : considered heating and used in mesalihs of horses. Natives suppose that infection and enchantment are prevented by its smoke.

Inderjau, इनदरजौ : Inderjan, इनदरजान : Nerium antidysentericum. The seeds are used, two kinds being sold, which though the product of the same species, differ in one being bitter and the other not so. The bark of this tree is the "codaga bark ;" but, is not used at Ajmeer. The tree is found in the Ajmeer district. The seeds are in long thin pods : the bitter seeds are used pounded to apply to the abdomen in colics from flatulency : are not given internally at Ajmeer. The other seeds are sweetish to the taste ; and used to excite venereal appetite ; for which purpose one tola is taken ; used also as a general corroborant. Four seers for one rupee.

Ingur, इंगुर : Shangruf, शंगरफ : Red Sulphuret of Mercury : Vermilion. Is brought from Pali and Delhie : two kinds ; one Chinese in powder in small packets ; the other in crystallized masses : is smoked in a hookah to salivate : one massee is inhaled in three days, and cures the venereal disease ; also is taken to cure impotence in a curious way : one tola of shangruf is wrapped up in a piece of cloth, and placed inside a cake of flour, called "buatie," made into a round mass, which is baked as usual ; the rag is removed and the bread is eaten ; this process is repeated for some days : the shangruf does not perceptibly diminish in quantity by the process : the natives foolishly imagine that the vapour of the vermilion affects the bread.

It is principally used in oil paintings, and as an ornament of caste : one seer costs from nine to twelve rupees.

Imli, इमली : Tamarindus Indica. The tree is abundant about Ajmeer : the fruit is much used in sherbets : considered both heating and cooling : used as a laxative.

Isquil, इसक़ील : Scilla (?) : Root of a species of Squill. One kind is found at Ajmeer ; but is never used : it is called "jungli piyaz."

Jaiphul, जैफल : Myristica moschata : Nutmeg. This spice is brought from Bombay viâ Pali : used as condiments, and in mesalihs of many kinds : costs nine rupees for one seer.

Jaiwutri, जैवतरी : Mace. Used in the same way : one seer for eleven rupees.

Jal-lakri, जललकरी : Billi-lotan, बील्लीलोटान : Valeriana (?) Officinalis. Plentiful about Ajmeer : the dried stalks are kept by "attars" on account of the scent : the root is not used : the effect of the plant on cats is well known to the natives.

Jangal, जंगाल : Subacetate of Copper : Verdigris. Is brought from Delhie and Agra, where it is made : comes also viâ Pali : used in painting ; and in some ointments in medicine. The Agra kind is three rupees, and the Pali kind two rupees per seer.

Jamal-gota, जमालगोटा : Croton tiglium. The seeds and roots are brought from Delhie : used as a common purge : the oil is a rubefacient : seeds costs one rupee per seer.

Jauwa-khar, जौवाखार. Ashes of barley leaves : considered cooling and diuretic : are employed in the "indri julabs" (which answer to our diuretics) ; one of these, is as follows ; jauwa khar, cubab chini, ilachi, rewand chini ; kulmee sora, misree, one tola of each : plenty of diluents drank on the top of the mixture.

Jadwar, जाद्वार : Zidwar, जीद्वार : Nirbusee, नीरबसी : Curcuma Zedoaria. Zedoary root, imported from Delhie : considered heating : used in medicine and medicinal diet : applied ground to boils to cause discussion : one seer costs two rupees.

Junj-bai-dustur, जंजबैद्सतर : Is true castor : imported viâ Delhie : is sold pure in its natural envelope : the natives have no idea of the beaver ; but, describe the castor as " the testicle of a small dog that swims in the sea or rivers ;" referring to the known habits of the beaver. The " attars" sometimes adulterate this substance very much : it is used as an aphrodisiac, especially by Mohammedans : one massee costs one rupee.

Juri-giri, जुरीगीरी : Duriya ke nariyal : Cocos Maldivica. The shell of the large nut of this tree comes from Bombay : is considered efficacious in checking vomiting : one seer for five rupees.

Jungli-long, जंगलीलोंग. The scentless and tasteless calyx of a flower from Mount Aboo ; in appearance very like the clove : considered heating : used in medicine : one seer for one rupee.

Jufa, Jufiah, जुफा : Croton Jufiah. The dried plant comes from Cabul and Odeypoor : considered heating, and used in cough mesalihs : one seer costs two rupees.

Huliabilsa, हलीबाबीलसा. An astringent seed brought from Delhie : given in diarrhœa : one seer costs four rupees.

Kath, कथ : the extract : } Acacia Catechu. The extract is used in
Khair, खर : the tree : } pawn ; and in medicine as an astringent.

Kala-mirich, कालामीरीच : Piper Nigrum : Black Pepper. Comes viâ Pali from Bombay ; one seer costs eleven annas.

Kaephul, कायफल : Rhododendron puniceum. A common tree on the lower ranges of the Himalaya hills : the bark, called kaephul is brought from Delhie and Mirzapoor, and is used as a rubefacient and sternutatory. I have found kaephul and pounded ginger, mixed, the best substance with which to rub cholera patients to promote re-action : one maund costs five rupees. The fresh flowers are pleasantly acid, and are eaten by the hill men to quench their thirst during the ascent of the hills : the flowers are also made into a jelly.

Kotki, कोटकी : Root of a plant found near water : it has neither taste nor scent : used in mesalihs.

Kalajira, कालाजीरा : Nigela Indica. Found growing about Ajmeer : the seed is used medicinally, and is heating and bitter : employed as an alexipharmic and in horse mesalihs.

Kesar, केसर: } Crocus sativus: Saffron. Brought from Bombay
Zafran, जफरान: } viâ Pali, and from Cashmeer viâ Beekaneer: is very dear: used as an emmenagogue: considered heating: given in mesalihs: two tolas cost one rupee.

Kakra singh, काकरासींग. Fruit of a tree brought from Harowtee: considered heating: given in coughs.

Kewanch, केवांच: Kooch, कुच: Dolichos pruriens. The plant grows about Ajmeer: the seed only is used by the natives: the hairs of the pods are applied to no use: in medicine the seed is considered aphrodisiac.

Kantala, कंटाला: Agave Cantula. The whole plant is considered heating, and used to excite perspiration in coughs.

Kulinjan, कुलींजान: Alpinia galanga. Root of the plant: is hot and stimulating: used in mesalihs: has a sweet scent: is put into bazar spirits to make it more intoxicating: two and a half seers for one rupee. The name also of the root of "piper betel."

Kankol mirich, कंकोलमीरीच. Seed of a plant brought from Bombay: is considered heating: used in prescriptions, and as a condiment: one seer for one rupee.

Kanoj, कनोज. Seed of a small tree brought from Pali and Delhie: considered heating and constipating: taken as a condiment, and also given as a medicine in diarrhœa: one seer for two rupees.

Katira ka gond, कातीराकागोंद: Katila ka gond: Sterculia urens. The white transparent gum of the kur tree: the tree is plentiful some distance from Ajmeer: tasteless and similar in property to tragacanth: swells exceedingly when placed in water; but does not dissolve: in medicine considered cooling and astringent, and given in "dai" and "luddoo."

Khar, खार: Suji, सजी. Partially fused ashes of a saline plant, brought from Sind viâ Beekaneer: prepared near the sea coast: about two hundred camel loads arrive every year: is chiefly impure soda: effloresces in the rains: contains also some deliquescent salts. Any quantity of good carbonate of soda might be made from this substance. It is sold all over India: at Ajmeer, one maund costs two and a half rupees. Is used in medicine, making glass choories, paper making, and dying with koosoom and indigo.

Khopra, खोप्रा: Nariyal, नारीयाल: Cocos nucifera. Cocoa-nuts are brought from Bombay: cost twenty-six rupees a maund: or, sixteen per rupee.

Kismis, Raisins ; cost sixteen rupees a maund.

Monuka, ditto without seeds ; cost twenty a maund.

Kuchila, कुचीला : Kuchla : Strychnos Nux Vomica. The seed of the fruit is brought from Delhie and the Mewar jungles : used in embrocations and eaten as an intoxicating substance in cold weather ; also taken as an aphrodisiac ; for the latter purpose, half a nut is first scorched, and then boiled in milk, which is thrown away, and the nut is eaten with sugar : is also boiled and eaten with rice in asthma : asthmatic people take to the extent of two nuts with great benefit :—given also internally in rheumatism and paralysis : is used in elephant and horse mesalihs : is sold four seers for a rupee.

Kasni ka jur, कासनीकाजर : Cichorium Endivia : Succory Root. Considered warm, stimulating, and febrifuge : given in " munjus," the diluent taken preparatory to purging : the seed is used in sherbets : is plentiful about Ajmeer.

Kakri ka bij, काकरीकाबीज : Kira, Khira : Cucumis Sativus. The seeds are used in infusions, as diluents, and in sherbets.

Karbuja ka bij, करबुजाकाबीज : Cucumis Melo.
Turbuja ka bij, तरबुजाकाबीज : Cucurbita Citrullus.
{ Seeds of both, used in the same way.

Kulfi, कुलफी. Seed of a small plant, both wild and cultivated about Ajmeer : considered refrigerant, and as such used in sherbets.

Kao, काव. Seed of a similar nature.

Koot, कुट : Costus Arabicus. Roots of the sweet and bitter costus plant : is brought from Delhie : hot and stimulating : said also to be narcotic when smoked, and formerly great quantities went to China for that purpose : given in medicine five or six massee are a dose.

Kupila, कपीला : Rottlera tinctoria. The dust from the capsule of the fruit is used : comes viâ Delhie : dyes silk yellow : alum is used as the mordant : considered in medicine as of a warm nature : also anthelmintic : given to children in " dai ;" three or four massee are a dose : used in ointments for herpetic eruptions : two and a half seers for one rupee.

Kusailoo, कसैलु : Kusaili. The bark of a small tree, wild about Ajmeer : is tasteless : given to lying-in women to clear the blood and create milk : from one to four pice's size form the dose in six or seven days.

Kaphur kachri, कापुरकचरी. A root from Delhie, having a sweet smell: used to make scents of: used in hair mesalihs: five seers for one rupee.

Kawul-gutti, कावलगट्टी: Nymphæa lotus. The seeds of the lotus; they are tasteless; but much used in medicine: mucilaginous: said to check vomiting: six massee are a dose: also eaten roasted as food.

Kesru, केसरू: Hursingar, हरसिंगार: Nyctanthes arbor tristis. The tubes of the corolla of the weeping nyctanthes, are brought from Mewar: considered heating: given in medicine, one tola a dose: used chiefly to dye yellow: two seers for one rupee.

Kilgutch, कीलगच: Katkaranja, कटकरांजा: Kutkaleja, Guilandina bonducella: Bezoari nut. The seed is very bitter: used very generally as tonic, febrifuge and deobstruent: common at Ajmeer: natives foolishly suppose the seed will cure a scorpion sting.

Kombhugras, कोमभगास: Root of a small plant from Delhie: tasteless; but is heating: one tola is given as a tonic or aphrodisiac.

Khatmi, खातमी. Althæa rosea (bura gul khairu): Hollyhock. The seed is considered cooling: in medicine one tola is given: the corollæ and pericarps when fresh are exceedingly mucilaginous and used in sherbets.

Khabaji, खाबाजी: Althæa alhugas (chhota gul khairu): Common Mallow. The seed is used in the same way.

Khub-kali, खबकेली: Khub-kala. The seed of the yellow fruit of a small tree about Ajmeer: very mucilaginous: considered refrigerant.

Kathir, काथीर: Ranga, रांगा: Tin. Comes from Bombay: the grey oxide is given as a tonic: used to colour glass, for choories, a white colour: one seer for one and a quarter rupee.

Kadu ka bij, कदुकाबीज: Tomra ka bij: Cucurbita lagenaria. Seeds of the bottle gourd; cooling and demulcent.

Kalmi sora, कलमीशोरा. Crystallized saltpetre, purified: considered refrigerant, and as such used in medicine. Best sort five rupees per maund; inferior sort four rupees.

Karu, कारू. Leaves of a climber found about Ajmeer: are bitter and used as febrifuge, and in mesalihs.

Kara chal, कड़ाछाल. Bark of a tree from Harowtee: used in mesalihs of camels and goats.

Kugnaj, कगनाज. Fruit of a climber from Delhie: cooling and astringent: used in mixed prescriptions.

Kirmali ka bij, कीरमालीकाबीज. Seed imported viâ Pali : considered stimulating.

Khas, Khuss-khuss, खसखस : Andropogon muricatum : Gandar grass. The fragrant root is used in tatties, and atr is extracted from them : used in sherbets.

Khairsar, खैरसार. Grains or pith from the wood of the catechu tree : considered as heating : used to promote perspiration : given in pawn leaves in coughs : one tola for eight annas.

Kala nimuk, कालानीमक : Black Salt. Is made by pounding together five seers of suji khar, two seers of dried anola fruit, and one maund of common salt, adding water, and boiling for some time : is considered to promote digestion : is much eaten : used in many mesalihs.

Kala dana, कालादाना : Ipomœa cœrulea (Convolvulus nil ?) Grows in the rains about Ajmeer : the seeds are much used, roasted and pounded as an effectual purge : one tola is taken by an adult as a dose : very cheap.

Long, लोंग : Eugenia caryophyllata : Cloves. Come from Bombay, Pali and Delhie : used as condiments and in mesalihs.

Lodh, लोध : Symplocos racemosa. The bark of the root is used : the tree is found in Rajpootanah ; but the root is imported from Delhie ; used in dying red ; also used in medicine : considered heating, and promotive of the secretions : used in mesalihs of animals : four seers for one rupee.

Lila tuta, Lila tota, Tootiya, तुतीया : Sulphate of copper. Is brought from Shekhawattie : is extracted at Ramgurh : used as an external application, and to cauterize ulcers ; but, is chiefly used in dying : two seers for one rupee : one maund costs from sixteen to twenty rupees.

Lila phool, लीलाफुल : Nymphæa cyanea. The plant is common in the Ajmeer and Poshkur lakes : the flowers are used medicinally : considered astringent and refrigerant.

Loban, लोबान : Styrax Benzoin : Gum Benjamin. Imported viâ Pali : used as a stimulant, and eaten in pawn leaves ; the "attars" sublime the benzoin acid very purely, and administer it as an aphrodisiac : one seer costs from two rupees to two and a half.

The gum resin of the Boswellia thurifera is also considered as "luban" by the community.

Laj-burd, लाजवरद : Lapis-lazuli. This is more or less pure ; imported from Bombay : considered refrigerant and astringent : also used in painting : one seer costs four rupees.

Laj-aloo, लाजआलु : Mimosa natans : Water Sensitive Plant. Found near Ajmeer : considered refrigerant and astringent : one seer for one rupee.

Long ka tel, लोंगकातेल. Oil of Cloves, from Bombay ; used as a stimulant and in scents : six tolas for one rupee.

Muraiti, मुरैटी : Abrus precatorius : Ghoonchi. Is found in abundance about the Ajmeer hills. The root is very similar to, and is sold for liquorice root : is considered astringent and refrigerant. The root should be dug up at the end of the rains.

Maida lakri, मैदालकरी. The bark of a large tree : is brought from Delhie and used in mesalihs.

Musli-sufaid, मुसलीसफेद : Asparagus sarmentosus. The root of the plant is brought from Kotah, and viâ Pali : considered of a warm nature and given in purges and mesalihs.

Musli-siyah, मुसलीसीयाह. Black root of similar shape and size, comes from Kotah : used in the same way : and considered stimulant and used as an aphrodisiac.

Mugrela, मगेला : Nigella (Indica ?) A black sweet-scented seed, especially when bruised : by being put among clothes or under carpets, insects are prevented from approaching or harbouring.

Mirchai, मीरचै. Another name for kala-dana.

Mooltani mattie, मुलतानीमटी. Soft yellow bole, common in Rajwarra ; used as a detergent, as an application to prickly heat (urticaria) ; it affords great relief, if left to dry on, and then washed off : used also in dying and distemper work : one maund costs one rupee.

Makoe, माकुइ. A species of sarsaparilla, common in the Dukhan : the berries are eatable : not used medicinally.

Mako, माको : Pulidun : Gurkhi : Solanum nigrum ; and Solanum rubrum. The dried black and red berries are indiscriminately sold as medicine : are also eaten fresh by the poor : the leaves are given in flatulency, and are eaten as a vegetable in dropsical swelling of the hands and feet ; are also pounded with ginger to rub the hands and feet : do not seem to be poisonous in India.

Methi, मेथी : Trigonella fœnumgræcum : Fœnugreek. The plant is much cultivated as a vegetable : the seeds used medicinally, are considered heating and carminative : are bitter : much used in mesalihs.

Malkhagni, मालखागनी : Celastrus paniculata. The seed is imported from Marwar, and Godwar : is considered sudorific, and generally heating : is bitter : the seed is swallowed whole in rheumatism : used in horse mesalihs.

Maror-phuli, मरोरफली : Helicteres isora : Screw-tree. This small tree grows at Ajmeer : the twisted pods are used : considered refrigerant and astringent, taken in curds in diarrhœa ; one pice's size is the dose.

Manjith, मांजीथ : Chhol-manjith : Rubia manjistha. The root of the manjith is largely imported from Kotah, Boondee and most parts of Rajwarra; also imported viâ Pali from Guzerat : is given in medicine as a febrifuge : used in many prescriptions : much used to dye lake colours and turkey red : the chhol-manjith is the best : one maund costs twenty rupees.

Main-phul, मैनफल : Vanguiera spinosa. The tree grows in Marwar : the dried fruit is used ; considered stimulating, and when given to cattle in the cold weather prevents their suffering from the cold : not given to mankind : three seers for one rupee.

Moordar sung, मुरदारसंग. Litharge is not made at Ajmeer, though there are lead mines : is brought from Delhie : used in ointments and in oil paintings : two seers for one rupee.

Murhatti ka jur, मरहाटीकाजर : Glycyrrhiza glabra : Liquorice-root. Comes from Delhie : used as a demulcent, and in compound prescriptions : two and a half seers for one rupee.

Rub-us-soos ; the extract of Liquorice. Comes from Bombay : considered cooling, and is eaten in coughs : one seer costs eight rupees.

Mainsal, मैनसाल. A mixed orange and yellow coloured sulphuret of arsenic : appears a mineral production, composed of orpiment and realgar : it is brought from Bombay : one massee is given internally in itch, mixed with sulphur and anola-phul, and boiled in milk ; is not taken alone : used also as a pigment : one seer costs two rupees.

Moongas, मुंगास. A middling-sized root, comes from Delhie : is tasteless ; occurs in the written prescriptions of hakims : is four to eight annas a tola.

Moonga ka jur, मुंगाकाजर. The root comes from Delhie : is very sweet : is taken mixed with "luddoo" in impotency and general debility.

Moti-buka, मोटीबुका. Small seed pearls from Bombay : are prescribed in impotency : one tola costs seven rupees.

Maju-phul, माजुफल : Gall nuts. Are imported viâ Pali : are used by women as an external application after child-birth, &c. &c : much used in dying : one seer costs one rupee eight annas.

Môr-pagi, मोरपागी. A small plant found about Ajmeer : used on child-birth occasions : has no taste.

Maida ka choor, मैदाकाचुर. Root of a plant brought from Delhie : has a sweet smell : considered refrigerant : one seer for one rupee four annas.

Mai-sutr-arabi, मैसटरआराबी. Blood which has congealed in the belly of a young camel ; after being overfed, the young camel is driven about violently, and then killed, when the blood is extracted ; is brought from Bombay and Delhie : supposed to benefit in impotency : one tola costs three rupees.

Mai-rubiya, मैरबीया. A dried fish brought from Delhie : considered good in impotency : four tolas for one rupee.

Mooli-khar, मुलीषार. Ashes of the radish leaves and root : considered refrigerant.

Mochras, मोचरास. The gum of the semal tree (Bombax heptaphyllum) : is a laxative and as such given to children.

Mûsk, mooshuk, मुसक : Musk (Moschus moschiferous). Is imported from the Himalayas : is not to be had good at Ajmeer : is much used and highly valued in impotency and as an emmenagogue ; also as a scent : costs twelve rupees for one tola.

Mus-abbâr ; the Arabic name for Aloes.

Naus-adar, नौसादार : Muriate of ammonia, imported from Delhie ; employed in embrocations : used in the arts : two seers for one rupee.

Nagkesur, नागकेसर : Mesua ferrea. The root of the tree is used : considered astringent and refrigerant : one tola is taken internally : is applied externally in cynanche.

Nak-chikara, नाकचीकाडा. The leaves of a small plant found about Ajmeer, also imported from Delhie : are very hot, and a good sternutatory : three massee are given in pills, as a dose in colic, which is said to be thus speedily relieved.

Nugar-motha, नगारमोथा: Cyperus pertenuis. Very common at Ajmeer : the root has a pleasant smell : used in hair mesalihs : also considered astringent and to check diarrhœa : one tola is given.

Nirmali ka bij, नीरमालीकाबीज : Strychnos potatorum. The seeds are imported viâ Pali : used to clear water, and to cure scorpion stings.

Nim-gilo, नीमगीलो : } Menispermum glabrum. A climber found
Gulancha, गुलांचा: } often on Neem trees; the whole plant is very bitter: the stem is chiefly used: six massee are given as a dose, with other ingredients in fevers. An extract called "giloysut" is prepared and much used.

Nar ka choor, नारकाचुर : Curcuma zerumbet. The white root, like huldee in shape, comes from Harowtee: has a strong smell and bitter taste: used as a rubefacient and in mesalihs: one seer for eight annas.

Oos-ara-rewand, उसाररेवांद : Stalagmitis gambogioides. Is real gamboge, and is imported viâ Pali: considered and used as a violent cathartic: the punsaris suppose it to be the extract of the Mirabilis jalapa root: the dose given is sixteen grains: one seer costs four rupees.

Ootingna ka bij, उटींगनकाबीज. Seeds of a small plant found about Ajmeer: are in taste bitter: considered aphrodisiac, and generally tonic.

Oost-kudoos, उसतकदुस. A sort of grass imported from Delhie: is given in "munjus" preparative to administering a purge: one seer for two and a half rupees.

Oodrooz, उद्रुज. A yellowish white gum, imported from Bombay: on being chewed, at first causes a sweet, then a bitter impression: used to apply to the forehead in head-aches: one seer for four rupees.

Ood-suleen, उद्सलीन. Short pods that are brought from Bombay: are considered as stimulant and antispasmodic: given in epilepsy and rheumatism: one tola is a dose. Native mediciners in their ideas connect rheumatism and epilepsy together, owing to the muscles being affected in both.

Oosbo-mugurwi, उसबोमगरवी. Said to be the root of the foreign Bur tree: considered heating; one seer costs ten or twelve rupees.

Oosuk, Ushuk, उसक : Gum ammoniac. Imported viâ Delhie: little used in medicine: sold by attars at two annas per tola.

Piplamôr, पीपलामोर : Piper longum. The root of the long-pepper plant: imported from Delhie: used as a condiment and carminative.

Pokhur-mool, पोखरमुल. The root of a plant imported from Delhie: considered heating: one "pice bhur" is taken in head-aches: used also in many prescriptions, and in mesalihs of animals.

Pattis, पाटीस : Cyperus inundatus. The plant is found near water:

the leaves are considered tonic, refrigerant and astringent: six massee are taken in diarrhœa.

Panri, पानरी. Leaves of a small plant imported from Bombay: considered refrigerant and to promote digestion; are sweet-scented, and used by attars: one seer costs one and a half rupees.

Padmak, पाद्मक. The wood of a tree from the Himalayas: considered to be refrigerant.

Pakhanbed, पाषनबेद. Root of a small plant imported viâ Pali: considered good in flatulent and other dyspeptic disorders: one seer for one rupee.

Para, पारा: Mercury. Comes viâ Pali: not taken internally by the natives: used in ointments: one seer costs eight rupees.

Patol, पाटोल. The seed of Luffa pentandria, used as a refrigerant.

Pust-burn, पस्तबरन. A grass from Delhie: considered cooling.

Papeeta, पापीटा: Papiya: Carica papaya. The dry fruit is kept, and used ground up in water to check vomiting.

Pharid-buti, फारीद्बुटी. A mucilaginous plant found at Ajmeer: used in sherbets.

Pakambri-nosadar, पकमबरीनोसादर: Artificial realgar. Comes from Delhie: used by fakeers: one tola for one rupee.

Phitkarie, फीटकारी: Alum. Comes from Sind, where it is made: about three hundred camel loads annually arrive: red alum is brought from Lahore: used in medicine as an astringent; but chiefly employed in dying: one maund for ten rupees.

Rai, राइ. Black and yellow mustard seed, eaten and used in mesalihs.

Raskapur, रासकापुर: Impure Calomel (Protochloride of Mercury). Comes from Bombay and Delhie: is given in eight grain doses to salivate in the venereal disease, and used in ointments: one seer costs eight rupees.

Rumi-mastungi, रुमीमास्टंगी: Pistachia lentiscus: Gum Mastic. Is brought from Pali and Delhie: is chewed by the natives as a tonic, and for the tooth-ache: is also given in medicine: one seer two rupees.

Rendi, रेंडी: Arandi: Irran: Palma christi. The castor oil seed is chiefly used to rub with in rheumatism, and to burn: sometimes is given as a purge.

Rewand kutai, रेवांद्कटै: Rheum palmatum. The rhubarb root is imported from Cabul: little used in purgative prescriptions: one seer for two rupees.

Rewand-chini, रेवांदचीनी. A root supposed by the punsaris to be that of the Mirabilis jalapa, brought from Delhie : used in purges, and as a diuretic.

g-mahec. Raikh-mai, रेखमै. Lacerta Scincus. The Scink found in the sand of rivers : imported dried viâ Delhie : considered aphrodisiac.

Rahusa ka tel : Rahusa grass oil ; used as a rubefacient : one seer costs fifteen rupees.

Sonth, सोंठ : Zingiber communis : Ginger. Comes dried, viâ Mirzapoor, Delhie and Rewarrie : used in embrocations ; but chiefly as a condiment : two seers for one rupee.

Siya-jira, सीयाजीरा : Carum Carui : Caraway seed. Brought from Cashmeer and Cabul : used as a carminative and condiment : also in mesalihs.

Sohaga, सोहागा : Borax. Comes from Delhie : sixteen rupees for one maund.

Satowar, साटोवार. Root of a climber found in the Ajmeer district : stimulating.

Sikakul, सीकाकल. Root like a carrot, brought from Cashmeer : used as an aphrodisiac. Colchicum Illyricum.

Soorinjan, सुरींजन : Hermodactylus. A root in appearance like the pignut : imported viâ Pali : is bitter and sweet in taste : used as an aphrodisiac.

Sumundr-sokh, समंदरसोष : Convolvulus argentaceus. A large creeper : the seed is used along with salep misri as an aphrodisiac : the half roasted leaves applied to the skin are escharotic : one tola of the seeds is a dose.

Sumundr-jug, समंदरजाग : Sumundr-phen. Bone of the cuttle fish : considered refrigerant : used in eye ointments : also in mesalihs.

Sumundr-phul, समंदरफल. A fruit imported viâ Delhie : considered carminative : used in mesalihs of elephants and horses.

Surma, सुरमा : Grey Sulphuret of Antimony. Imported viâ Pali from Bombay and Lahore : used externally, chiefly to the eyes ; especially in the eye pigment so named : one maund costs forty rupees.

Sufaid-surma, सफैदसुरमा. Crystallized rhomboidal carbonate of lime : used as a dentifrice.

Somp ka jur, सोमपकाजर. Root of a Rajpootanah plant, considered heating and febrifuge : one ingredient of " munjus."

Soa ka bij, सोआकाबीज : Anethum soa : Fennel seed. Used as carminative in food and mesalihs.

Surali, सराली. Seed of a small Ajmeer bush : are astringent and refrigerant.

Sunna maki, सन्नामाकी : Cassia senna. Senna leaves, imported viâ Pali and Delhie: much used as a purge: two seers for one rupee.

Salep-misri, सलेपमीसरी : Orchis mascula: Salep root. Imported from Cabul and viâ Bombay: eaten as restorative and aphrodisiac: the natives have the usual absurd ideas regarding it: the best sells for one rupee per tola.

Sats-arila, सटसरीला : Flowers of the Kaiphul tree (Rhododendron puniceum). Have a pleasant scent: come from the Himalaya hills: used in hair mesalihs.

Sungtaras, संगतरास : Panpak: Steatile. Found in the hills about Ajmeer; and brought from Bombay: women eat it in "luddoo:" used in ointments.

Sisa, सीसा : Sisu: Lead. The ore is found and worked in the hills at Ajmeer: the vitrified oxide is used in eye ointments: white and red lead are also used in ointments.

Sambhal-khar, सांभलखार : Arsenious acid. Brought viâ Pali: there are three kinds, white (sankia), yellow (zurd), and red (soorkh): is used in ointments as a counter-irritant: fakeers burn it in a certain mixture, which they then eat, and they declare that in consequence their naked bodies do not suffer from the cold in the winter: one seer costs six rupees.

Sunkmuniya, संकमुनीया : Convolvulus scammonia. Scammony is imported viâ Pali: used as a purge: four massee are given: one seer costs four rupees.

Sathara, सथारा : Origanum (?) Sp. Leaves of a plant found about Ajmeer, are considered febrifuge and refrigerant.

Singia moora: सींगीयामुरा : Haldia moora. Roots that come mixed with haldi: they are acrid and poisonous, and are carefully separated.

Sanda, सांडा : A sort of Lizard. It is distilled, and the product applied, by Mohammedans, to the penis: the reptile is also eaten as an aphrodisiac.

Sugandh-kokla, सुगंधकोकला. A small sweet-scented berry used in making scents, and as a refrigerant.

Salburni, सालबरनी. A small plant from Delhie, considered stimulant.

Sufaid-chirmi, सफेदचीरमी : Sufaid goonchi: Soorookh goonchi. Red and white seeds of the varieties of Abrus precatorius: are bitter and reckoned stimulating: supposed to be poisonous.

Suja-balud, सुजाबालद. Pods of a plant from the Himalayas: are astringent: one rupee per seer.

Sung surmaiyi, संगसुरमैयी. A concretion from the head of a fish; comes from Delhie: used as an aphrodisiac: sold at eight annas a tola.

Sung misri, संगमीसरी. A red and white stone, imported viâ Pali: is used as an aphrodisiac: one tola for one anna.

Satr-sowa, सतरसोवा: Myrtus communis: Myrtle leaves, are eaten with black pepper to cure emissions of semen that occur from debility.

Sirkist, सीरकीसट: Manna, in white grains. Considered cooling: used as a laxative: one seer for fourteen rupees.

Sirka, सीरका: Vinegar. Made at Ajmeer, sold by "attars:" considered refrigerant: used in embrocations: three seers per rupee.

Semal ka phool, सेमलकाफुल: Flowers of the Bombax heptaphyllum. Considered refrigerant.

Sowan-muki, सावनमकी: Iron pyrites. Comes from Bombay: considered refrigerant, and used in itch ointments: two rupees a seer.

Sahat, साहत: Honey. From Mewar and Kotah: much used in medicine, especially for coughs: two seers per rupee.

Sung-diryao, संगदरीयाव. An impure and weak Nitro-muriatic acid, made by attars, by mixing equal parts of alum, nitre and salt with a little water in an earthen gurra, and distilling: an acid fluid comes over that is applied to cure herpetic eruptions.

Isquil. Scilla maritima. Is not imported into Ajmeer.

Taz, ताज: Outside bark of the cinnamon tree, used in mesalihs,

Tal makhana, तालमाखाना: The seed of the plant comes from Shekhawattee: is stimulant: used in general debility; but chiefly as an aphrodisiac.

Tukhm-mullunga, तुखम-मलंगा: A very mucilaginous seed, imported from Delhie: considered cooling, demulcent, and much used in sherbets.

Tas ka jur, तासकाजर: Root of a climber found at Ajmeer: is bitter and purgative: one pice bhur purges fifteen times or more.

Tej-pat, तेजपाट. Leaves of the bay laurel, from the Himalaya hills: used in food: employed in mesalihs of animals.

Tugur, तगर: Tiraimun: Uparoon: Tabernæmontana coronaria. The sweet-scented wood and root are imported from Delhie and Kotah: considered and used as a stimulant; but chiefly used in scents.

Tiriya pharka, तीरीयाफारका: Treea pharook. A black extract (most likely extract of henbane) of a narcotic odour: imported viâ Bombay, carefully packed in small tin boxes: is a powerful stimulant, and is given in a sort of convulsive disorder called "seet" (catalepsy): one tola costs six or eight rupees.

Tukm-kurpus, तुषमकरपस. Seed of a plant from Delhie, astringent and stimulating: given in flatulent indigestion: two rupees a seer.

Tukhm-gandah, तुषमगंधना. A seed from Delhie, considered astringent.

Tambra-bij, तामबरबीज. Seed of a small plant from Harowtee: stimulant.

Turanj-bij, तुरंजबीज. Saccharine grains imported from Bombay: are used in purges: one seer costs ten rupees.

Aloes Wood. Aquilaria Agallocha.

Ugur, अागर. A sweet-scented wood imported viâ Bombay: considered refrigerant; but chiefly used in worshipping.

Umbl-bhaiti, आमबलभैटो: Ambl-bhaiti; Oxalis carniculata. The stem of this plant is imported from Delhie: very sour: used to cure flatulent indigestion.

Zira-sufaid, जीरासफैद: Cuminum cyminum. Cumin seed. Plentiful about Ajmeer: much used in food and mesalihs.

Zaffron, जाफरोन: Saffron: Kesur.

Zowanie, जोवानी. Seed of a small cultivated plant: promotes digestion.

Indian Medical Science at a very low ebb.

From this selection, a tolerably clear impression of the vile, depressed state of native medicine may be ascertained: the great inquiry among the medicines being still for objects to cause an increase of salacity.

All the remedies of any importance are still retained, or have been long rejected from our pharmacopœias.

Many Europeans in India are still of opinion that native hakims and bueds are often superior in knowledge to, are at any rate are in possession of secrets unknown to, regular practitioners: I will only instance one among the articles of the native materia medica, than which none is more vaunted, the har or harra, considered to possess wonderful general deobstruent and purgative qualities, &c. &c. while those who thus belaud it, are apparently not aware that this is the chebulic myrobalan (Terminalia chebula) of our pharmacopœias of the sixteenth century and long since deservedly neglected.

I have known the opinion to which I allude, to have been carried so far, as to cause an officer to allow, if not to encourage, the men under his command to seek medical aid from the native hakims and bueds of the neighbouring town; a course which can only throw undeserved discredit on our profession, and serve to foster the native prejudices against us.

I trust that if any such gentleman honours by a casual perusal this digest of native practice, which the hakims and bueds themselves will allow to be learned in *their* ideas, he may have his prejudices removed.

Longevity. No instances of excessive longevity came under my observation; but, from inquiry I am of opinion that a large number of the inhabitants attain a good old age. Opium eating, and the use of bhang and spirituous liquors, unless when carried to great excess, do not seem to shorten life. The small-pox has the greatest effect in depressing longevity, by carrying off thousands, both in infancy, and from eight to twenty years of age. To this latter cause, the small population may be mainly attributed.

Zoology. I am not aware of any animal peculiar to this district: the common animals are domesticated, among which the camels and bullocks are superior, as are also a few of the horses. In the plains and hills the usual game is met with, often abundantly.

Amongst the game birds, the bustard may be deserving of notice, as being more common than elsewhere.

Amongst the fishes, the trout, plentiful in the Bunas river, is deserving of remark.

To arrange a scientific account of the animals of this district, I am not prepared.

Organic Remains. The strata of the district being of a primitive nature in general, and rarely secondary, no organic remains have as yet been discovered, either of mammalia, aves, pisces, molluscæ or amphibia.

Geology. The general character of the district in this respect is of the primary, or plutonic hypogene, and metamorphic hypogene formation, as is evinced by the soil of the plains, the debris of the hills, and the hills themselves. The latter are in appearance often serrate, and generally abrupt; and though not volcanic, the jagged ridges give them often that appearance. This serrate aspect seems owing to the hardness of the rock composing the hills, the sharp points of which, uninjured by the attrition of water still point to the skies, while less compact portions, in which these have been imbedded, have been long since washed away. Primary Rocks.

By far the greater part of these hills are schistose, and very rarely purely slaty.

The minerals composing them are often abruptly and most heterogeneously mixed together: large masses of nearly pure quartz and hornblende occur in contact: amorphous and glassy felspar, sandstone, or carbonate of lime, are found in juxta-position with granite, and amidst the latter large portions of felspar, quartz and mica, in distinct pieces, united together only by one side, are often to be seen: quartz with schorl, mica schist, hornblende schist, and quartz rock, frequently met with, stratified in close vicinity.

The term hypogene (produced below) used by Lyell, is well applied to the Ajmeer stratified rocks, which have evidently undergone a very high temperature below the surface. To be convinced of this a person has only to examine the elevated, generally western face of the schist strata, especially the mica schist; in some places portions of the otherwise horizontal strata, may be observed twisted and bent in an extraordinary manner, and still to remain quite unbroken: 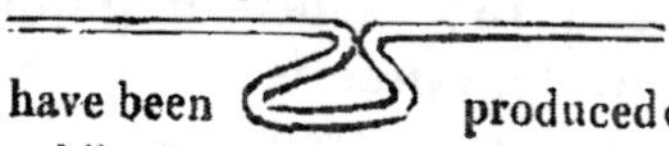 : an effect which could only have been produced on this hard brittle substance while it was in a state of semi-fusion, during some convulsion of nature, at a great depth, and under enormous pressure.

As in other hypogenic formations, so in these, a similar want of arrangement is manifest: no doubt owing to the violent convulsions of the earth, which first depressed the strata of schist which had been deposited horizontally by water, to a great depth; where after exposure to a semi-vitrifying heat, these were at a subsequent period as roughly elevated in the present heterogeneous appearance,

Hence, the mica schist, hornblende schist, quartz rock, felspar rock, hypogenic limestone, shew a variable order of super-position.

In general the highest points of the hills are of quartz rock, sometimes of a pure white; but, generally of a rust colour from the iron contained; and by far the greatest portions of the Ajmeer rocks, those of the Aravulli range and of Rajpootanah generally, except in the puttâr or table-land, are of this description. The lowest part reached in digging the deepest wells are also white quartz or dark granite.

The same granite is also found at the base of some of the hills, and protrudes through the surface of the plain, in several places near Ajmeer and in the district.

The granite of Ajmeer, does not consist of mica felspar and quartz, which have been generally considered as the sole minerals essential to constitute granite; a distinction too limited for practical purposes.

The first and most common kind of granite at Ajmeer is found at the foot of the Satpoora range of hills near Ajmeer and also opposite to the magazine, and appears to underlie the schistose strata throughout the country. It is fine-grained, and is composed of distinct transparent grains of quartz, separated by green hornblende in minute portions; the colour of the rock is dark grey; it is very hard and the fracture is irregular. In this distinct granite, neither mica nor felspar, is seen. This granite is again found abundantly at Shapoora (a hundred miles from Ajmeer) under the surface of the plain; of the same composition, with the exception of containing numerous grains of schorl. Near Shapoora some very ancient temples built of this stone are to be seen.

The second kind of granite is found in rolled masses and broken pieces among the Ajmeer hills, a portion of some of which are formed of it, and others in the district altogether consist of this rock; which is of a pinkish colour, composed chiefly of pink felspar, with quartz and grains of hornblende: the term syenite has been applied to this granite; but with great impropriety, and inconvenience to mineralogists, as it is evidently a pure granite. The conical hill of Sukrani is entirely composed of huge boulders of this granite, externally blackened by time; and around the base lie large round masses, which by a hard blow with a hammer break off in regular peelings, evidently indicating that they have been suddenly cooled at one period from a semi-fluid state.

The first kind underlies the other rocks throughout a great part of Rajpootanah: the second kind contributes to form the hills of the primary class in this district, in the Aravulli range, and in some of the hills of Boondee and Kotah.

Common serpentine of a dull liver colour, occurs in abundance near Sambhur, and is sometimes used to build with: it contains magnesia so abundantly that after exposure to a white heat sometime, it will slake with water like quick-lime, giving out great heat, and forming a cement; I have not met with serpentine elsewhere in Rajpootanah.

Gneis has not been met with pure: the schist of Kishengurh and some other places, consists of silica, mica, hornblende and felspar: it is extracted in considerable slabs, which are coloured grey by the quantity of hornblende contained. The cleavage in the small is irregular into broad scales, and the slabs are easily fractured: this therefore is not properly gneis; but, hornblende schst.

Micaceous schist is very abundant in this district, and also in Boondee: it forms large portions of hills: the strata are inclined from west to east and are sometimes twisted, yet unbroken: the Ajmeer mica schist is a very beautiful rock, and being abundant is generally used to build with: in many portions the silex is quite transparent: this schist is too brittle to be taken out in large slabs.

Hornblende schist is also very common: it is most pure near the Ana-sagur ghaut, where it forms part of a hill, and is there composed of hornblende and felspar only. A large portion of the Ajmeer and Kishengurh hills is of this rock, more or less slaty, composed of mica, hornblende, felspar and quartz, in large irregular scales.

Argillaceous schist does not occur in the Ajmeer district; but is very abundant in Boondee and Kotah: in the bed of the Ghora Parchâr nuddee in Boondee, near Nogong, excellent roofing slate is abundant.

Primary limestone crystallized, occurs in the Ajmeer district, in fissures or thin strata: one kind is very hard, pure white, and consists of large crystals; but is only used to burn into plaster, as it will not work evenly: another kind of a finer grain is also made into lime, being of an inferior colour. Limestone is also found composing portions of hills in Boondee, and from the marble, "kolhoos" or sugar and oil mills are made. Mukrani, in Marwar, produces the most beautiful crystalline marble and calcareous alabaster, which have been extracted during ages; it there lies in strata beneath and perpendicular to the surface.

Compact felspar is abundant in the district, and varies from white glassy to pinkish brown, and occurs in large masses: it is often mixed with quartz.

These form the great mass of the rocks of Rajpootanah, of an eminently primary character.

Secondary Rocks.

Of the secondary class of rocks, I believe, the lowest red sandstone does not occur, except at Kharee in Beekaneer; but variegated sandstone forms the top of a hill near Ajmeer, under the name of "Gogra ka bāta," and, is elsewhere, very abundant near Sambhur, where some is curiously variegated, and at Jaepoor: it is also universal below the surface, throughout Northern Marwar, all Beekaneer and Jessulmeer, and through great part of Southern Boondee, and all Kotah; and with white sandstone (or freestone) forms the "puttâr" or table-land of Kotah and Mewar; overlying the quartz rock of the bed of the Chumbul.

Shale, rapidly decomposing, forms many of the hills and eminences in the Kotah territory, and is also met with in Boondee.

Secondary yellow limestone of a beautiful kind occurs at Jessulmeer, and also a kind of "breccia," formed of minute vermicular yellow portions in a case of red ochre; and secondary concrete limestone is burnt for lime at Ajmeer.

Overlying rocks are also to be found; but, what has been said will be sufficient to shew, that far to the north of Ajmeer the secondary character prevails, while at Ajmeer and to the south and west, the primary character is maintained throughout.

Trap Rocks and Soils.

In this district, volcanic or trap rocks do not exist. I am aware that formerly the hornblende schist (of felspar and hornblende) would have been considered a trap rock; but it is evident that this schist at Ajmeer, is of the metamorphic hypogenic character, equally with the micaceous schist.

Werner restricted the term trap to rocks principally characterized by the presence of hornblende and black iron clay; yet, stated that in the oldest or primitive trap, no iron clay occurred. The presence of hornblende, and felspar, augite and felspar would have been more comprehensive and accurate: though either of these two combinations cannot, from composition alone, be designated trap, which is now universally allowed to be of igneous origin.

Near Bansrore in Mewar, the bed of the Chumbul is deeply cut down through soft white sandstone forming falls of considerable height, the sandstone has been cut by the powerful vortices into round hollows, called "choolis" (i. e. cooking places), in the bottoms of which round masses of basalt are abundantly found: these are washed down in the floods from Malwa: they are called "rori" or "rolli," and are worshipped as Mahadeva's and much valued. This basalt fuses easily before the blowpipe.

It is perhaps a curious fact that the natives are aware that these stone, are of igneous origin, and hence they are held sacred to Mahadeva.

Near Shapoora (two hundred miles distant from Bansrore)

I saw a pair of basaltic stones, supposed by the ignorant priests, to have been "dhoolkies," or drums of Mahadeva, which are held sacred.

At the "Chumbul ka choolis," near Bansrore, no basaltic rocks exist in the neighbouring hills, which with nearly the whole country and bed of the river, are of sandstone, except at the lowest part where the quartzose rock has been exposed in the bed of the river.

It has been customary to attribute the origin of the stiff black soil of Kotah, Malwa, Hoshungabad, &c. to the decomposition of basaltic rocks: especially from the circumstance of zeolites and calcedony being frequently found in the soil; but I here beg to remark that I have been led by circumstances to conclude, that the much more probable origin of these soils, has been the decomposition of argillaceous shale, which can still be often viewed in a state of rapid decomposition, especially at one small hill near the Chumbul, below Bansrore, composed of argillaceous and hornblende shale; the soil at the foot of the hill, and for a long way round was composed of the debris, which though still granular at the base of the hill, was at a certain distance, a rich, strong black soil, exactly like the Hoshungabad soil. At the latter place no basalt is discernible anywhere; but, the portions of sandstone that protrude above the surface shew the most clear marks of having been surrounded to a considerable height by a softer material that has gradually left them denuded. The same is observed at the foot of the Vindhya range.

One curious fact may be here worthy of mention, and that is, that on the Ajmeer hills, portions of rock composed of quartz, mica, and felspar, repeatedly occur in distinct pieces, united on one side, in such just proportions, that could they be triturated and re-united by cement or fused by heat, the result would be excellent granite.

Mineralogy.

Class I. Order I. Gems.

Prismatic corundum or chrysoberyl, is found among the Tora hills near Rajmahal on the Bunas, in irregular rolled pieces, small and generally of a light green colour: these stones are considered by the natives as emeralds, and pass under the name of "punna;" but the natives are aware that they are still softer than the real emerald of India, (which is generally green-coloured sapphire). Prismatic Corundum.

Schorl occurs abundantly in the vicinity of Ajmeer and elsewhere in the district: very beautiful crystals of it are found imbedded in milk-white quartz: minute crystals also occur very abundantly in some of the granite: it is also found in massive broken and rolled pieces near the abandoned copper mine near Ajmeer; and has been mistaken for lucullite (or black marble): the crystals become electric by heating. Schorl.

Chrysolite is found in the form of small pebbles of a pale green colour and semi-transparent, in the bed of the nullah near the same mine: it is not however sufficiently coloured or transparent to be of any great beauty: it melts with borax into a greenish mass. Chrysolite.

Garnets are to be found in abundance in beds of various nullahs, that flow from the schistose hills: they are found generally small; but are sometimes of considerable size; their form is usually a rhomboidal dodecahedron: they are of a claret red colour, and more or less transparent. I seldom found any of a sufficient degree of purity to be cut into gems. Garnets.

Quartz is very abundant, and chiefly common quartz; rock crystal, milk quartz, and calcedony are also met with frequently: onyx of a coarse kind is not uncommon in detached pieces; and hornstone is found in the same way. Quartz.

Cornelian, rolled or broken, pebbles are found in the beds of some nullahs; both of white and reddish veined varieties; but very impure. Cornelion.

Heliotrope or bloodstone is found in small detached irregular pieces in the beds of some nullahs, generally of a green colour, and seldom having red spots. Heliotrope.

Jasper is rarely found in rolled pieces, among the sand of the nullahs; it is of a dull liver colour. Jasper.

Common porphyritic jasper, of a dull liver colour, forms extensive hills in Boondee, as especially shewn in the beds of nullahs between Boondee and Tolera river.

Jasper agates occur in small fragments in the beds of the Bunas and other rivers.

Mocha stones of a beautiful kind are found in the bed of the Chumbul.

Moss Agates. Agates of a common kind are frequently met with on the plains: fortification agates are also found occasionally: moss agates of a small size are found in the bed of the Bunas.

Opal. Common opal is sometimes found massive, in broken pieces of a milk white colour, very brittle and translucent: at the base of the Sirinugur hills.

Those enumerated are all of the order of gems, that have come under my own notice, in the Rajpootanah territory; but from the geological nature of the country it is most probable that many other species of the gems may be discovered.

Order II. ORDER II. *Spar.*—Prehuite of the foliated kind has been found in hornblende near Ajmeer; but has not come under my own observation.

Spars. Zeolite. Zeolites of the figure of an acute double-sided pyramid, with crystals of a hexahedral form, are found rarely among the debris of the Ajmeer hills. To the south in the black soil of Kotah, Boondee and other places, zeolites are very commonly met with, of the figure of eight-sided double pyramids, united by the base with dodecahedral prisms: these latter zeolites were formerly imbedded, along with the numerous reniform calcedonies in the argillaceous schist, the decomposition of which has formed the present soil.

Lapis Lazuli. Azure stone or lapis lazuli is said to be found massive, with iron pyrites, amongst the Ajmeer hills, especially the Nag-puhar range: this stone is sold by all "attars" both as a medicine and as a pigment: though found in the district, it is also imported into Ajmeer from Bombay: the native name is "laj-burd."

Calaite. Calaite, or mineral turquoise, is said to be found amongst the hills in the district, and also at Ramgurh in Shekawattie:

it is generally of a sky-blue colour, and is used to set in common rings: it is called by the natives "peeroza," the Persian name.

Felspar of almost every variety is abundant. Glassy felspar is common: a large mass of it protrudes through the ground, opposite the Dowlutbagh, on the road to the Anasagur bund. Felspar.

Common felspar, chiefly pink and white, occurs abundantly in separate pieces; but chiefly combined with quartz in different proportions; and as an ingredient in granite, and schist.

Compact felspar is found in fissures, and in rolled pieces in nullahs among the hills.

Alumina, in combination with carbonic acid, is imported in the shape of small distinct concretions, like a seed in appearance, under the name of "Huzrutzahoor," from Cabul, and used in medicine. I am aware that it has been supposed that carbonate of alumina cannot exist in the dry state, but that this is carbonate of alumina is evident, by dissolving the stone in diluted nitric acid; the solution is rapidly formed with great effervescence, and on adding pure ammonia to the saturated solution, alumina is copiously precipitated, and re-dissolved on adding an excess of ammonia. Clay Family. Aluminite.

Common clay occurs of a light yellow colour in many places below the surface. A very stiff yellow loam containing free soda, is found in the interstices of the quartz rock of the Ajmeer hills, especially in the lead mine of Taraghur: the same loam is laid bare in beds in digging tanks and wells in some places in the district; and is abundant below the surface in Boondee, Kotah and Mewar. Common Clay.

Potter's clay of a coarse kind and bluish grey colour is found in sufficient abundance for manufacturing purposes, in most parts of Rajpootanah, and is generally a very recent deposit. Potters Clay.

Clay shale of a greyish black colour, mixed with green hornblende slate, rapidly decomposing, is abundant in Boondee, Kotah and Mewar, where the debris forms a stiff black soil. Clay Shale.

Clay Stone. Clay stone occurs massive, of a light brownish red colour, forming large rocky beds in the nullahs between Boondee and Kotah.

Adhesive Slate. Adhesive slate of a light straw colour forms part of the bank of the Chumbul at Bansrore; it adheres strongly to the tongue.

Clay Slate. Clay slate of a good roofing kind is common in Boondee, though not used for this purpose. Every kind of clay slate is to be found in Boondee.

Yellow Bole. Yellow earth of a slaty texture is met with in the district in digging some wells; but not of a superior quality. Throughout Beekaneer and towards Mooltan, it forms large substrata, and is exported all over India under the name of "Mooltanie mittie." This earth is commonly used as a detergent, especially to clean the hair. Made into a paste with water it is applied to the skin when covered with articaria or prickly heat, and allowed to dry on, and affords relief from the irritation, probably by breaking universally the small vesicles. while contracting in drying.

Kyanite. Prismatic kyanite is found abundantly with felspar, in the quartz rock of the Rajgurh hills in the Ajmeer district: the crystals are small and of inferior colour, and not large enough to be worked for any purpose. Surgeon Hezekiah Clarke discovered this mineral at Rajgurh.

Hornblende. Hornblende occurs imbedded of a dark olive green colour, massive, with a two fold cleavage, in veins in the hill of mica, quartz and hornblende, near the Ana-sagur.

Hornblende also forms the granite below the schist mixed with transparent granular quartz: and is an ingredient in the syenite granite, and in hornblende schist, both pure and mixed.

Hornblende slate is mixed with the clay shale in Boondee, &c. and also occurs distinctly in Boondee, of a dark green colour.

Asbestus. Irregular pieces of common asbestus are frequently to be met with amongst the debris of the hills: they are generally of a light greenish grey colour, and the fibres are twisted.

Amianthus, or flexible asbestus is also found, though it has not come under my own observation.

Ligneous asbestus is sometimes found in small broken pieces.

Prismatoidal nugite, epidote, occurs in small granular concretions in the syenitic granite, and felspar and quartz rock at Ajmeer. Augite.

ORDER III. *Mica.*—Of this order, white antimony is said to be found in the Ajmeer hills: and is sold in the bazars by the punsaris under the name of "sufaid soorma;" but I have never been able to meet with a pure specimen: those sold as such having been large rhomboidal crystals of carbonate of lime. Order III. Mica.

Common mica, called "abrukh" by the natives, is a most abundant mineral in the Ajmeer district; forming with quartz large hills of mica schist; mica in tables is very common, united to quartz and felspar. In some places vary large tables of talc can be extracted. It also occurs in nests of considerable magnitude. Common Mica.

Common chlorite occurs in veins of the mica schist. Chlorite.

Green earth, of a peculiar kind, occurs in the cavities, and at the edges of the carbonate of lime, in perpendicular fissures of the schist; but it is not of a bright colour, or in sufficient quantity to use.

Talc varieties occur, distinguished only from mica by want of elasticity; i. e. if bent, the plates do not resiliate, which those of mica do. Talc.

Indurated talc slate occurs amongst the schistose rocks. Steatite.

Steatile or soap stone is found in veins in some parts of the clay slate of the Boondee territory. The natives call it "sung-turas" (or stone-cutter).

Figure stone or agalmatolite, though not found in the district, is imported from Cabul as a medicine, supposed aphrodisiac. It is brought in considerable pieces along with "huzrutzahoor" and "junj bai dustar," &c. &c. Figure Stone.

Clay slate, though included by Jameson under this order, has already been mentioned under the head of the clay family.

Nephrite. Nephrite is for sale sometimes fashioned into the handles of daggers or swords: it is brought from a distance.

Serpentine. Common serpentine is found near Sambhar, in abundance, of a light liver colour, it is often curiously marked.

Fullers Earth. Fuller's earth is found near Ajmeer in fissures of quartz and schistose rocks, with carbonate of lime.

Order IV. ORDER IV. *Malachite.*—Common copper green ore crysocolla, occurs in small veins in brown copper ore, in quartz rock, mica and hornblende schist, at the old copper mine near the Grogra hills.

Malachite. Compact malachite is also found in small pieces at the same old mine.

Brown Copper. Brown copper ore surrounds the malachite veins.

These ores (carbonates of copper) were formerly worked for the copper they contained: the copper however was in too small a quantity to yield profit to the extracters. Ammonia, poured on the small portions of ore found, instantly assumes a deep blue colour; the ore therefore though small in quantity is tolerably rich.

Order VI. ORDER VI. *Baryte.*—Of this order tri-prismatic lead spar, or sulphate of lead, is found along with galena, very rarely, in the lead mine of Taraghur at Ajmeer; it is of a greyish white colour, and crystallized in small prisms: it is attached to milk quartz, surrounded by yellow sandy loam: the quantity is too small to work as an ore.

Baryte. Sulphate of Lead.

Barytes. Carbonate of barytes and sulphate of barytes I have met with in rolled pieces in the nullahs, exactly similar in appearance to those found in the Pentland hills in Scotland.

Order VII. Haloide. ORDER VII. *Haloide.*—Foliated granular limestone occurs near Ajmeer, in veins in mica and other schists and quartz rock: it is of a beautiful colour; but cannot be worked as the crystals are too large, and chip out in working; it is therefore only burnt into plaster.

Granular Lime Stone. Another variety occurs, less pure, in considerable beds in hornblende schistose rocks, at Kekree and other places in the district, and is also burnt into lime.

Most beautiful white marble and cretaceous alabaster is dug out in slabs below the surface of the plain at Makrani in Marwar. The quarries have been worked for ages. Some is perfectly pure white, semi-transparent and fine-grained.

Common compact limestone occurs in Boondee in the hills near Naogong: the stone is a sort of marble, being grey, and traversed by white crystalline grains. This limestone overlies the clay slate. It is not burnt into lime; but sugar-mills are made of it. Compact LimeStone.

Fine-grained yellow compact limestone is found at Jessulmeer, forming a considerable hill.

A beautiful variety is also found at Jessulmeer, formed of small yellow vermicular cretaceous particles, thickly set in a base of red ochre: the limestone can be speedily removed by an acid, leaving the porous red iron clay behind. The tomb of Aurungzebe, at Aurungabad in the Dukhun, is made of an exactly similar stone.

Agaric mineral, or rock milk, is very abundant in hollows in the soil and in fissures in rocks of Ajmeer and to the south-west. It is generally composed of fine white dusty particles of pure carbonate of lime: and also in small semi-crystalline concretions in loam or marl, near Ajmeer. The latter is dug out and constantly used as a cement, becoming very adhesive with water. It is known by the names of "moorum" or "moorur." From repeated experiments this is evidently pure carbonate of lime;—and with the exception of the grains being crystalline, the mixed earth does not differ from the "moorum" of other parts of India. Agaric Mineral. Moorum.

Tufaceous limestone, or calc-tuffa, occurs in the hills to the south-west of Ajmeer: it is of recent formation and is of a spongy texture, containing no impressions of plants, &c. it is burnt into common lime that is used at Ajmeer. This only differs from the calc-tuffa of Hosungabad, in containing no impressions of plants, &c. Tufaceous LimeStone.

Travertin limestone is abundant in the bed of the Tolera nuddee near Boondee: it is in horizontal layers, hard and compact, regular, and more or less recent; and is deposited over the hard clay stone rock of the bed of the river. Travertine.

Lucullite. Lucullite (or black marble) has never been met with by me in this district or other parts of Rajwarra. Massive schorl has been mistaken for this.

Marl. Marl is very abundant in many places under the sand, or light sandy loam, in this district and in Jaepoor, especially near Doodoo; it is called "pandole," and is only used to cover the walls of native houses. The soil might be much improved by its use.

Gypsum. Sulphate of lime, though said to have been found in the Ajmeer district, has never come under my observation, notwithstanding a rather diligent search.

Class II. Order I. Fossil Salts. CLASS II. ORDER I. *Fossil Salts.*—Vast quantities of lake salt in cubicular crystals are extracted at Sambhur chiefly, and also at various other smaller lakes or "sirs" in Marwar and Beekaneer, and from the Looni or salt river.

Green Vitriol. Green vitriol, or sulphate of iron in an impure state, is prepared at Ramgurh in Shekawattie, from the refuse of the copper and iron pyrites of the mines: it is sold cheap under the name of "sada kusees."

Blue Vitriol. Blue vitriol, or sulphate of copper, occurs native in the soil at Ramgurh in Shekawattie; but is chiefly prepared by exposing to air and moisture, the copper pyrites of the mines, for a considerable time, and then lixiviating.

Glauber's Salts. Glauber's salt, or sulphate of soda, is found in the Sambhur lake in considerable abundance, and can be obtained in crystals, after the removal of the chloride of sodium.

Saltpetre. Prismatic nitre, or nitrate of potash, is abundantly produced on the surface of some portions of the soil, formed of decomposed mica and felspar, and covered with old bones, &c. it is collected by the "kharols," purified and exported.

Soda. Natron, or carbonate of soda, is very abundant as a white efflorescence on the surface of the low grounds: it is also found in some lakes in Beekaneer: it is removed with the earth and is called "reeah:" it is used either native, or purified, by the dhobies, and in dying. Any quantity of fine soda might be obtained in this district.

Borax. Borax; tincal; sohaga: sub-borate of soda, is said to be produced in Beekaneer.

Class.III. Order.I. Native Metals.

CLASS III. ORDER I. *Native Metals.*—Grains of gold are said to have been found formerly in the beds of the Looni and Khari rivers.

Silver.

Native silver is also said to have been found in the mica schist in making a well in the city of Ajmeer: this well was attempted to be examined by Captain Dixon; but the flow of water was too great, and could not be mastered by the means employed.

It is very probable that, in the extensive tracts of mica schist, quartz rock, granite, syenitic granite, &c. &c. very valuable minerals may still be found.

Copper.

Native copper has been found rarely in small pieces attached to the rock: this metal also occurs native, in the Shekawattie mines.

Order.II. Ores. Copper and Iron Ores.

ORDER II. *Ores.*—Copper ore in the form of sulphuret is chiefly abundant in Ramgurh in Shekawattie: near Ajmeer the carbonate of copper is found in small veins, and in connexion with ores of iron.

Iron ore of excellent quality is abundant in the Ajmeer district; large irregular masses occur in the beds of the nullahs: at Jehazghur, on the borders of the district, excellent siliceous iron ore is worked on a considerable scale: the iron extracted is of a good soft quality. In the Ajmeer district any quantity of iron may be extracted from the iron ores of the hills and plains.

Specular iron ore is found in irregular rolled pieces in the nullahs.

Ochry red iron ore, or red ochre, is found abundantly near Beekaneer: it is called "geeroo."

Ochry red clay, or red chalk, iron ore, is also extracted under the same name.

Order.III. Pyrites.

ORDER III. *Pyrites.*—Iron and copper pyrites have already been mentioned.

Order.IV. Glance. Galena.

ORDER IV. *Glance.*—Galena or lead glance is the ore of lead, imbedded in quartz rock, that is now worked in the mine of Taraghur at Ajmeer: the lead extracted is considerable in quantity and pure, containing no trace of silver. The mine is worked by the government, and the lead might be manufactured into articles that would yield a more profitable return, than the pure lead.

Antimony. Antimony glance, "kala soormu," or sulphuret of antimony, is also, though rarely, found among the lead ore in the same mine.

Such are the few ores of metals that have been discovered in Rajpootanah. An extensive research amongst the primitive hills, especially the Aravulli range, would, I have no doubt, lead to the discovery of valuable metalliferous and other veins. The fact of the mines being a royal prerogative, under the classification of "an, dan, kan," certainly leads to suppose that mines of value were worked at former now forgotten periods.

Some account of the botany of Ajmeer, Kotah and other places, adjacent.

MONANDRIA MONOGYNIA.

Canna Indica: Indian Shot. Hind: Ukulkurra. Sans: Survajuya. Two varieties are cultivated as ornamental in gardens at Ajmeer, one with scarlet, the other with yellow flowers. The punsaris keep the root by the name of ukulkurra: it is considered acrid and stimulating.

Phrynium Dichotomum. Hind: Pattee-patee. Is cultivated in some gardens at Kotah, as rare and ornamental.

Hedychium Coronarium. Garland flower. Hind: Goruknatha. Cultivated as a fragrant flower in gardens at Kotah. A yellow variety is also met with.

Kæmpferia Galanga: Galangala. Hind: Sans: Chundramoolika. Common in gardens. The root is kept by punsaris as sweet-scented, stimulant and carminative.

Kæmpferia Rotunda: Round-rooted Galangala. Hind: Bhoo-chumpa. Cultivated at Kotah, &c. as a flower. The root is often sold by the punsaris as zedoary root.

Curcuma Zerumbet: Zedoary. Hind: Kuchoora. Cultivated as a flower; blossoming without leaves, in the hot winds.

Curcuma Zedoaria: Broad-leaved Turmeric. Hind: Bun-Huldi. Arab: Zadwar. Cultivated in the Rajah's gardens at Kotah. The roots are kept by the punsaris, who import them from Chittagong, where these plants are indigenous. The root is reckoned a perfume, and in medicine is used as stimulant and carminative, and applied externally as discutient. The red powder (called abeer and phag) used at the Holi is made, in some places, of this root, mixed with sapan-wood powder.

Curcuma Leucorrhiza: White-rooted Turmeric. Hind: Thikoor, Tikor. Is found in the jungles of Kotah and Mewar, &c. The root yields a fine white farina like arrow-root; and this is sold by the punsaris as "tikor," and used as an article of sick diet.

Curcuma Longa: Common Turmeric. Hind: Huldi. Is cultivated in Kotah and Mewar.

Zingiber Officinalis: Common Ginger. Hind: Udhruk (when green); Sonth (when dry). Is cultivated about Ajmeer; but is chiefly imported dried.

Costus Speciosus }
Costus Arabicus } Costus. Hind: Keoo, Koot. The plant is still to be met with in the black soil, during the rains. Formerly the plant was largely cultivated, and exported to China, where it was smoked, as opium is now, before the poppy was largely cultivated in India. A preserve is made of the root of costus speciosus.

Alpinia Galangala: Alpinia Galangale. Hind: Kulinjen. I have not met with the plant; but the root is kept by the punsaris, and is said to be produced in Kotah: it is used as a scent, and in medicine and mesalihs: it is also put into bazar spirit to render the liquor more intoxicating.

Alpinia Alhugas: Ceylon Alpinia. Hind: Sans: Taruka, Tara. Found in the marshy parts of the black soil of the Kotah jungle.

Alpinia Nutans: Nodding-flowered Alpinia. Beng: Poonag-Chumpa. Cultivated in gardens: was brought by myself from Tonk to Ajmeer: the flowers are beautiful, and the whole plant is fragrant like the cardamom: the seeds do not ripen.

DIANDRIA MONOGYNIA.

Nyctanthes Arbor Tristis: Weeping Nyctanthes. Hind: Hursingar. Cultivated as a rare flower: the blossoms are very fragrant: the tubes of the corollæ are used, under the name of "kesru," to die buff or orange colour. This plant is very abundant wild at the foot of the Vindhya range, where the green tough stalks are used to make large grain baskets of.

Jasminum Zambac: Arabian Double Jasmine. Hind: Motiya. Cultivated abundantly at Ajmeer.

The largest double variety is called "hazarea mogra," and was brought to Ajmeer, from Cawnpoor, by me.

The single "motiya" is also cultivated.

Two beautiful varieties are also cultivated, called "satha," with single and double flowers, which have the odour of fine green tea. The double kind was brought from Lucknow. These are probably the Jasminum Scandens of Willdenow.

Jasminum Pubescens: Downy-leaved Jasmine. Hind: Koond. Cultivated as a flower, and is very ornamental; but, it is curious that the flowers of Ajmeer (a light soil) have no scent, while at Hoshungabad (a stiff black soil) the flowers in the mornings are highly odoriferous.

Jasminum Arborescens: Tree-like Jasmine. Hind: Munun-manus. A beautiful large fragrant flowered species, cultivated at Ajmeer.

Jasminum Auriculatum: Auriculated Jasmine. Hind: Juhi. A small sweet flowered species, much cultivated at Ajmeer.

Jasminum Chrysanthemum or Revolutum: Curled-flowered yellow Jasmine. Hind: Pela-Chambeli. Cultivated, and is a very free flowerer and highly ornamental.

Jasminum Grandiflorum: Catalonian Jasmine. Hind: Chambeli, Jati. Much cultivated at Ajmeer for the flowers.

Eranthemum Pulchellum: Nervose Eranthemum. Hind: Gool-sham. Found under the shade of trees in the Kotah jungles.

Justicia Picta: Painted Justicia. Hind: Soorookh-Vasooka. In the Fakeer's gardens, near the Bund at Ajmeer.

Justicia Adhatoda: Malabar Nut Justicia. Hind: Alusa Bakus, Vasooka. Grows abundantly wild: is used medicinally.

Justicia Nasuta: White-flowering Justicia. Hind: Juhi-pana. Found in the native gardens as a flower. The flowers are sold along with those of jasmine; and the rest is used in medicine as an excitant.

Justicia Ghandurussa: Willow-leaved Justicia. Hind: Jugut-mundun. Cultivated in the Kotah gardens: also found in Fakeer's gardens: used medicinally.

Justicia Verticillata: Erect Justicia. Hind: Kustoola. Found in the Kotah jungles.

Gratiola Serrata: Notched Hyssop. Hind: Bhoomia-neem. Grows wild during the rains: used as a bitter by the poor.

Salvia Bengalensis: Bengal Sage. Hind: Shisti. Cultivated in Europeans' gardens at Ajmeer: the Hindoos think this a very impure plant.

TRIGYNIA.

Piper Betel: Betel Pepper. Hind: Pawn; Tamboola; Tamboli. Is cultivated in some gardens: especially in Kotah and Mewar.

TRIANDRIA MONOGYNIA.

Valeriana Jatamansi: Spikenard. Valerian. Hind: Jul-lakri; Jutamansi; Billi-lotan. Is very common near water during the rains. The stems are used chiefly as a scent. The effect of the plant on cats is well known, and hence the name billi-lotan, or "cat tumbler."

Hippocratea Arborea: Tree-like Hippocratea. Hind: Katha-puhariya. Found in Kotah hill jungles.

Iris Chinensis: Chinese Iris. Cultivated as a flower in Europeans' gardens.

Morea Chinensis: Chinese Morea. Hind: Dusbi-Chandi. Cultivated as a flower.

Commelina Bengalensis: Bengal Spider Wort. Hind: Kanshira; Kunuraka. Grows wild in low ground during the rainy season. The leaves are sometimes used as a vegetable by the poor.

Commelina Salicifolia: Willow-leaved Spider Wort. Hind: Panee-kanshira. Grows wild.

Commelina Nana: Dwarf Spider Wort. Grows wild.

Commelina Nudiflora: Naked-flowered Spider Wort. Hind: Kandali. Grows wild.

Kyllingia Monocephala: One-headed Kyllingia. Common in low grounds. The root is sweet-scented: used and named as zedoary, "nirbishee."

Cyperus Rotundus: Round-stemmed Cyperus. Hind: Mootha. Very common in low grounds. The small fragrant tubers are used in washing the hair.

There are several other varieties: one of the most common is "naga-mootha," the root of which is used in the same way.

Scirpus Incurvatus: Club Rush.

Scirpus Articulatus: Jointed Club Rush. Hind: Putputi-cheelka. Both grow in standing water at Ajmeer.

Scirpus Atropurpureus. On wet sandy land.

Scirpus Schœnoides. Amongst bushes in pasture ground. Hind: Moormoori.

And several other species.

Penicellaria Spicata: Bull Rush. Hind: Pathera. Grows abundantly in the Poshkar lake and the Sarasvati nuddee.

Cenchrus Lappaceus: Bur Cenchrus. Hind: Boor; Bruit. Found abundantly on dry land: is very annoying to the naked feet.

Saccharum Cylindricum: Lagurus Cylindrica: Cylindric Hare's-tail grass. Hind: Oola. Grows on the plains, and flowers early in the rains.

Saccharum Spontaneum : Thatching grass. Hind : Kus ; Kush ; Kāgără. Very abundant in the plains ; where the blossom in the rains has a beautiful silvery appearance. Brooms are made of the culms, and string of the leaves, and the whole to thatch with.

Saccharum Officinarum : Sugar-cane. Hind : Ik ; Ak ; Ook ; Gunna ; Pounda ; Rusāla ; Sētha. The small white variety called "boora" is cultivated in this district for sugar, by irrigation : in Kotah and Boondee this variety does not require irrigation, and this is the case generally in the black soil. The long jointed red variety is cultivated by the malees in the gardens, and is sold in the bazars and eaten in great quantities by all who can afford to buy it.

Saccharum Procerum : Lofty Saccharum. Sirkunda ; Sārkara. Very abundant every where on the sandy ridges and plains, where water is not very far from the surface. The lower parts of the culms, called sirkunda, are made into outside cheeks for door ways, &c. ; the upper parts of the culms, called sirkee, are made into excellent neat and cheap mats, much used in thatching, &c. the floral leaves are made into "moonj," by separating the fibres, by beating the leaves ; this is very much used to make string and rope.

Saccharum Sara. : ——. Hind : Sur ; Shura ; Goondra. Common in the plains. The culms are finer and stronger than sirkunda, and are used to make arrows of, in preference to the other species when obtainable. The species of saccharum are often confounded by the natives.

Saccharum Moonja : Moonj Saccharum. Hind : Surpat ; Surpata. Common at Ajmeer in the valleys and very abundant along with the saccharum procerum, near Jaepoor. The best moonj is made from the floral leaves of this plant ; and the best sirkee from the culms. The plant is distinguished from saccharum procerum by the height, which is inferior, the fineness of the culm and narrowness of the leaves.

Andropogon Serratus: Serrate Andropogon. Hind: Khura; Khurrur; Jeemota. Grows in moist places in the plains: is considered the best grass at Ajmeer to preserve for cattle.

Andropogon Aciculatus: Needle-like Andropogon. Hind: Soorwulla; Soorwul; Spear-grass. Sans: Shunkinee. Abundant in barren land, troublesome to the feet of those who walk among it; eaten by cattle when other grass is not to be had.

The common names of this variety are "lampa" and "cho-ra-kanta."

A larger variety known solely as "soorwul" is an excellent grass for cattle.

Andropogon Muricatus: Sharp pointed Andropogon. Hind: Gandar; Garrar, the plant; khuss-khuss, the root. Abundant in the black alluvial soil of tanks and jheels. The fragrant root is much used for tatties, &c.; and the leaves to thatch with.

Andropogon Bicolor: Black Joar. Hind: Kala Joar. Is cultivated in some places.

Andropogon Sorghum: Indian Millet. (Sorghum Vulgare.) Polygamia Monœcia (?). Hind: Joar. Extensively cultivated in rather better ground than the bujra will thrive in.

Andropogon Schœnanthus: Lemon Grass. Hind: Ghundabena. Cultivated in gardens.

And other species.

Digynia.

Paspalum Scrobiculatum: Punctured Paspalum. Hind: Kodo; Kodă ka choul. Cultivated in light barren soil, in Kotah and Mewar, during the rains. The small white grain is palatable.

Paspalum Kora. Hind: Kodū. Cultivated and used in the same way.

These grains eaten newly gathered, sometimes owing to some disease of the plant, have a most extraordinary effect on the poor natives who consume them: affecting them with all varieties of delirium: the people of a whole village thus affected form an extraordinary spectacle.

Panicum Spicatum: Holcus Spicatus: Panic Grass Millet. Hind: Bujra. Very universally cultivated, as a rain crop, being the staple grain crop of the more barren parts of Rajpootanah. Twenty stalks from one seed are common, even in very poor ground.

Panicum Dactylon: Agrostis Linearis: Doob Grass. Hind: Doob; Doobra. Very abundant every where, where there is the least moisture. The best grass for all cattle.

Panicum Ciliare: Ciliated Panic Grass. Hind: Makurjalee; Kur-makra. Found in the fields near water-courses.

Panicum Brizoides: Quaking Panic Grass. Hind: Odagāss. Grows in tufts in most places, that are not saline.

Panicum Hirsutum: Hairy Panic Grass. Hind: Jul-ganti. Grows near water.

Panicum Italicum: a kind of Millet. Hind: Kungoo; Kungnee. Cultivated like kodū, during the rains; is eaten by the poor in Kotah and Mewar, in the hilly districts.

Panicum Frumentaceum: Corn-like Panic Grass. Hind: Shama. Cultivated by the poor to the south of Ajmeer, as a grain, on a small scale.

Panicum Miliaceum: Millet. Hind: Chēēna. Cultivated in the poor parts of Kotah.

Festuca Triflora: Three-flowered Fescue Grass. Hind: Bunjooa. Common near gardens and edges of fields; eaten by cattle.

Milium Filiforme: Thread-like Milium. Hind: Kankajuriya. Grows with doob grass.

Agrostis Tenacissima: Tenacious Bent Grass. Grows in tufts in marly ground.

Holcus ———. A species of holcus, called Raj-gira (or royal seed), is cultivated on a small scale in Kotah for Maharatta consumption. The grain is very small and smooth, and is very agreeable to the palate, eaten parched. The Maharatta brahmuns eat this only on fast days.

Chloris Tenella : Tender Chloris.
Chloris Montana : Mountain Chloris. } Found in the damp grounds near the Ana-sagur.

Chloris Barbata : Bearded Chloris. Common in the plains.

Poa Bifaria : Two-rowed Poa. Common in the plains.

Poa Cynosuroides : Dog's tail Meadow Grass. Hind : Doob-gāss ; Darbha. Sans : Cusa ; Koosha. Grows on dry pasture lands : used in religious ceremonies : cattle will not eat it.

Other species of Poa are abundant.

Eleusine Egyptica : Egyptian Eleusine. Hind : Makara-jŭli. Grows in pasture grounds, and is eaten by cattle.

Eleusine Coracana : Thick-stalked Eleusine. Hind : Nut-chanee (the grain), Murooa, the plant : sometimes cultivated for the seed.

Arundo Karka : Hooka Pipe Reed. Hind : Nurkut ; Nūda. Abundant in hedges and gardens, near water. Of the leaves, the "durma" mats are made. Elephant Grass.

Rottbœllia Glabra : Smooth Rottbœllia. Hind : Burroo ; Kowrēna : Job. A tall grass, growing near water ; found near the Bunas river.

Hordeum Hexastichon : Winter Barley. Hind : Jao ; Jowa. This is the staple grain of the rubbee crop.

Triticum Æstivum : Summer Wheat.
Triticum Hybernum : Winter Wheat. } Hind : Gehoon. Are cultivated during the cold seasons, wherever the soil is sufficiently good.

Both wheat and barley are irrigated.

Trigynia.

Mollugo Pentaphylla : Five-leaved Mollugo. Hind : Khet-papra. A common weed in gardens.

Mollugo Triphylla : Three-leaved Mollugo. Hind : Jul-papra. A common weed.

Mollugo Verticillata : Whorled Mollugo. A common weed in gardens.

Amongst others of this class, the "roos" or "răhūsa" grass, is common in the hills ; but is put to no use.

This grass appears to be a species of "festuca," and from the colour might be called "Festuca fusca." The distilled oil is imported and held in high estimation.

Tetrandria Monogynia.

Spermacoce Hispida : Hairy Button Weed. Found in flower in the cultivated fields during the rains.

Rubia Manjistha : Indian Madder. Hind : Manjistha; Munjeet; Chol-munjeet. Much cultivated in Boondee, Kotah and Mewar, in black loam : the root is largely exported. A beautiful crimson lake colour is dyed with it in Rajpootanah.

Ixora Bandhooka : ———. Hind : Bandhooka; Ruktŭka. In the Kotah gardens and jungles; and is a beautiful bush, covered with numerous scarlet flowers all the year, and would be very ornamental in our gardens.

Ixora Parviflora : Small-flowered Ixora. Hind : Gundhul; Runghun; Jilpai, (at Kotah.) On the banks and near talaos at Kotah; the flowers are very sweetly scented, and the tree blossoms in the hot weather; would form a very fit ornament for gardens and pleasure grounds.

Salvadora Persica : Persian Salvadora. Hind : Peelow; Jhal. Very common tree in Ajmeer and Marwar. The bright green of the leaves is very refreshing to the eye, as the tree grows in very barren places; it is generally semi-recumbent on the ground, and affords little shade. The leaves and bark are very acrid, smelling very strongly of cresses : the freshly pounded bark of the root is an active epispastic, not known as such to the natives of Ajmeer; but, I have employed it so successfully.

Plantago Ishpaghula : Indian Plantain. Hind : Isabgūl; Uspagool. Cultivated in gardens for the seeds, which are used as demulcent and astringent.

Cissus Vitiginea. Vine-leaved Cissus. Hind : Guali-lata. Found in the Kotah hill forests.

Cissus Quadrangularis : Square-stalked Cissus. Hind : Harjora. A common climber in the Kotah hill jungles : found also on the Nag-puhar at Ajmeer.

Oldenlandia Biflora: Two-flowered Indian Madder. Hind: Purputee; Papra. Appears in moist ground in the rainy season.

Ammania Vesicatoria: Blistering Ammania. Hind: Daudmaree. Found in the malees' gardens near the hedges in the rains: the pounded leaves are applied by the natives to herpetic eruptions.

Trapa Bispinosa: Two-horned Water Caltrops. Hind: Singhara. Much cultivated in tanks during the rains. The seed is much eaten boiled or roasted.

Santalum Album: } White and Bastard Sandal Wood.
Santalum Myrtifolium: } Hind: Sundul; Chundun. Cultivated at Kotah and near Jaepoor, for the wood which is used to form the funeral pyres of the great. The tree is not allowed to grow large enough to render the wood very odoriferous. The foliage would be ornamental to our garden grounds.

Digynia.

Cuscuta Reflexa: Twisted Dodder. Hind: Huldi-luta. A parasite found on bushes during the cold season.

Pŏtamogèton Indicum: Indian Pond Weed. Found on the marshy side of the Poshkur lake.

Pentandria Monogynia.

Heliotropium Indicum: Indian Turnsole. Hind: Hattisoor. Common wild in gardens and fields.

Borago Zeylanica: Ceylon Borage. Hind: Belatti-kulpa. Cultivated in some gardens as a flower.

Menyanthes Indica: Indian Buckbean. Hind: Bura-chooli. In standing water at Ajmeer and Poshkur.

Plumbago Zeylanica: Cingalese Leadwort. Hind: Chitruka; Chitruk; Lall chitruk. Found near the hedges of the gardens. The root is very acrid, and is sold by the punsaris as an epispastic.

Plumbago Rosea. Hind: Lall Chitruk.

Convolvulus Gangeticus: Pink-flowered Convolvulus. Cultivated as a flower, and also abundantly wild; with several varieties of different colours.

Convolvulus Argentaceus : Silver-leaved Convolvulus. Hind : Sumunder-sokh. Cultivated as a flower : the leaves and juice of the plant are acrid, and applied by the natives to stimulate sores.

Convolvulus Bi-color : Two-coloured Convolvulus. Hind : Zurd-kulmi. A yellow and buff-flowered Convolvulus, cultivated in gardens.

Convolvulus Turpethum : Turbith-root Convolvulus. Hind: Turbad ; Teoree. On the hills amongst the "Thuar" during the rains. The bark of the root is used as a purge, by the natives, and is called "turbad."

Convolvulus Arvensis : Field Bind Weed. Common in the fields, and exactly resembles the English kind.

Convolvulus Dianæ (?) : Moonlight Convolvulus. Hind : Chand. Cultivated in gardens ; the large fragrant white flowers open in the evening and fade in the morning.

Convolvulus Hirsutus : Hairy Convolvulus. Found during the rains.

Convolvulus Digitatus : Finger-leaved Convolvulus. Common in the hedges during the rains, with purple and blue flowers.

Convolvulus Repens : Creeping Convolvulus. Hind : Kulmi Shak. Cultivated on the dried-up bed of the Anasagur ; the stalks are used as a vegetable.

Convolvulus Batatus : Sweet Potatoe. Hind : Sakur-kund. Both red and white are largely cultivated, and are superior.

Lettsomia Argentea. Same as Convolvulus Argentea.

Ipomœa Grandiflora. Same as Convolvulus Dianæ.

Ipomœa Cærulea : Sky-blue Ipomœa. Hind : Neel-kulmi ; Kala-dana. Wild in the hedges about Ajmeer. The seeds called kala-dana are kept by the punsaris, and are much employed as a purge ; but reckoned very irregular in operation.

Ipomœa Phœnicea : Scarlet Ipomœa. Common in hedges and gardens during the rains.

Ipomœa Quamoclit : Wing-leaved Ipomœa, White and Crimson. Hind : Lal-kamluta (the crimson), Swetakamluta (the white). Pers: Isŭk-pŭcha (love's ringlets). Both cultivated as highly ornamental.

Ipomœa Pes Tigridis: Tiger's Foot Ipomœa. Hind: Kumra; Pora-batul. Very common in the rains and after, every where in Rajpootanah.

A most beautiful extensive perennial Ipomœa is to be seen at Raj-gurh and in the residents' garden at Ajmeer, generally called the Malabar creeper; it has bright yellow flowers and glabrous palmate leaves. This species seems to agree with the Ipomœa Tuberosa of the West Indies, only this has no scent. This plant extends to an immense length, and affords a very close shade.

Nauclea Cadamba. Hind: Kadam. Plentiful in Kotah, Boondee and Mewar; rare in Ajmeer. The wood is soft and fine-grained like satin-wood. The flowers are fragrant and are called "kurun-phool." This tree would be highly ornamental in "compounds," along with the bukain and neem.

Rondeletia Tinctoria: Dye-wood Rondeletia. Hind: Tooralodh. The tree grows in the Kotah and Mewar jungles; the bark is used in dying red.

Vanguiera Spinosa: Thorny Vanguiera. Hind: Muyna; Mainphul. Grows in the Kotah and Mewar jungles; the dried berries are given to cattle, and the fresh berries are sometimes eaten by the inhabitants.

Morinda Citrifolia: Broad-leaved Morinda. Hind: Bŭra-āl. This tree is common in Kotah and Boondee. The flowers have a very sweet scent, and the tree would be ornamental and thrive well in compounds.

Morinda Tinctoria: Dye-root Morinda. Hind: Al; Ach. Largely cultivated at Boondee, Kotah and Mewar. The root is extensively exported as a red dye: the colour is fixed with alum. The plant is not allowed to shoot up into a bush; but is dug up the third year after planting. The flowers are very fragrant. Of the large plant the berry is eaten.

The wood of all the species is beautiful, hard and durable; and excellent for gun stocks.

Morinda Multiflora, and other species are also found.

Datura Fastuosa: Purple Thorn Apple. Hind: Kala Dhatura. Wild and cultivated; both single and double varieties. The double flowers are beautiful and fragrant. The seeds are kept by the punsaris, under the name of "kŭnŭk-bij." They are given to intoxicate. The whole dried plant is excellent when smoked in asthma.

Datura Metel: White or Downy Thorn Apple. Hind: Dhatura. Very common everywhere as a weed; there are several varieties.

A beautiful large double, yellow-flowered, fragrant species, is cultivated in gardens at Ajmeer; and is easily raised without deterioration from the seed.

Physalis Flexuosa: Flexuose Winter Cherry. Hind: Isgandha; Asgandh. Common at Ajmeer; the roots are sold by punsaris, and are considered stimulating and diaphoretic.

Physalis Peruviana: Cape Gooseberry. Hind: Tepurya. Cultivated in gardens for the fruit.

Solanum Lycopersicum: Love Apple. Hind: Belatti-baigan. Cultivated in gardens, and thrives well at Ajmeer.

Solanum Rubrum: Red Nightshade. Hind: Makoe. A common weed. The leaves are sometimes eaten as a vegetable by the poor; the red berries are also eaten raw, and kept dried by the punsaris.

Solanum Nigrum: Black Nightshade. Hind: Kala Makoe. A common weed also. Neither are at all poisonous in India. The natives suppose they are diuretic.

Solanum Melongena: Egg Plant. Hind: Baigan; Brinjal. Several varieties are largely cultivated as a vegetable.

Solanum Jacquini: Jacquini's Nightshade. Hind: Kanthakaree. This very common weed is put to no use.

Solanum Diffusum: Wild Baigan. Hind: Junglee-baigan. Grows wild in many places; is put to no use.

Capsicum Purpureum: Purple Capsicum. Hind: Kala-gach-mirich. Is cultivated and sold in the bazars.

Capsicum Annuum: Annual Capsicum. Cultivated in European gardens.

Capsicum Frutescens: Fruitful Capsicum. Hind: Lal-gach-mirich, and Pila gach-mirich. Both red and yellow varieties are cultivated.

Capsicum Minimum: Bird Chilly; or Cayenne Capsicum. Hind: Dhan-lunka-mirich. Cultivated as a small shrub.

Strychnos Nux Vomica: Vomic Nut-tree. Hind: Kuchla. Grows in the Kotah jungles, near Mookundurra: the seed is exported.

Strychnos Potatorum: Clearing Nut-tree. Hind: Nirmŭlee. Grows wild in Kotah and Mewar. The seeds are not used to clear water with in Rajpootanah.

Cordia Latifolia: Broad-leaved Cordia. Hind: Bura Lusora. This tree is common at Ajmeer. The fruit is eaten. Of the bark "phaleetas" or slow matches are made. This tree is hardy and ornamental, and would do well in compounds, along with other trees.

Cordia Myxa: Smooth-leaved Cordia. Hind: Lusora. Also common at Ajmeer; the glutinous fruit of both is eaten.

Cordia Serrata: Saw-leaved Cordia. Hind: Gab; Gad; Gondori. Common in hedges at Ajmeer. The small gummy berries are eaten as a fruit by the poor.

The wood of each of these species is excellent.

Tectona Grandis: Teak. Hind: Sagoon. A small species of this tree grows in Kotah and Mewar.

Zizyphus Jujuba: Jujube-tree. Hind: Byer. A large fruited grafted variety, is cultivated about Ajmeer, and very much so near Jaepoor. The wild tree is common and the wood much used.

Zizyphus Microphylla: Small-leaved Jujube. A very common small bush, universally used to form hedges with.

And other species; one of which is semi-scandent.

Cedrela Toona: Toon-tree. Hind: Toon. Is cultivated in the gardens at Kotah.

Mangifera Indica: Mangoe-tree. Hind: Am. Cultivated wherever the soil allows: the fruit is generally inferior: the best comes to Ajmeer from Kotah and Jaepoor.

Impatiens Balsamina: Balsam. Hind: Gool-mendi. Cultivated, and abundant wild.

Musa Paradisiaca: Common Plantain. Hind: Kāla. Cultivated at Ajmeer; but are generally inferior.

The banana, or musa sapientum, is not cultivated in Rajpootanah.

Achyranthes Aspera: Prickly Chaff-flower. Hind: Chirchiria. This is a very common weed, especially in gardens.

Celosia Cristata: Crested Cock's-comb. Hind: Lál and Peela Moorgh-kes. Both white and yellow varieties are cultivated in gardens.

Celosia Argentea: White Cock's-comb. Hind: Sufaid Moorgh-kes; Sĭrwărie. Double variety cultivated. The single variety is very common in the rains in cultivated fields, both white and pink, and cattle eat the plants, especially buffaloes.

Celosia Ceruna: Drooping Cock's-comb. Cultivated as a flower.

Carissa Carandas: Jasmine-flowered Carissa; Caronda. Hind: Karonda. Cultivated for the fruit at Ajmeer. The plant grows abundantly wild in the Kotah jungles, and in March and April fills the air with the fragrance of its blossom. This plant forms beautiful and impassible hedges.

Ophioxylon Serpentinum. Hind: Chota-chand. Cultivated in the gardens at Kotah; but the inhabitants do not believe in its reputed virtues.

Gardenia Latifolia: Broad-leaved Gardenia. Hind: Pāpŭră. Grows wild in the moist Kotah jungles, and is also cultivated in gardens.

Gardenia Gummifera: Gummy Gardenia. Grows wild on the hills in the Kotah jungles; the leaves and unopened blossoms, being shrouded at the point in pure fragrant gum resin.

Gardenia Florida: Cape Jasmine. Hind: Gool-chand; Gundhuraj. Both double and single varieties are commonly cultivated in gardens at Ajmeer; the foliage is beautiful, and the pure white double blossoms are elegant and fragrant.

Vinca Rosea: Rosy Periwinkle. Hind: Suda-phool; Goolfering. Very plentiful in gardens at Ajmeer.

Nerium Odorum: Sweet-scented Oleander. Hind: Kanel. Plentiful and very beautiful at Ajmeer. The single white is called sufaid-kurpud; the single rose-coloured, lal-kurpud; and the beautiful large double rose variety is called pudma-kurpud.

Nerium Coccinæum: Scarlet Oleander. Hind: Soorookh-kanel. Common in gardens at Ajmeer, and it is highly ornamental.

Wrightia Antidysenterica. Hind: Inderjau; Inderjan. Found in the hill jungles of Kotah and Mewar; there are two varieties. The seeds are used medicinally by the natives. This tree would do well in compounds.

Allamanda Cathartica: Purging Allamanda. Hind: Peela-kanel. Cultivated in gardens for its bright green foliage and bright yellow blossoms. The whole plant is full of an acrid milky juice.

Plumieria Acuminata: Acuminated Plumieria. Hind: Gool-achin. Common in gardens, and grows to a large size in time. The blossoms are beautiful and very fragrant, and the whole tree very ornamental, and easily cultivated.

Vitis Indica: Indian Grape. Hind: Ungoor. Several varieties are cultivated at Ajmeer and Poshkur, and the fruit is very superior.

Tabernæmontana Persicariafolia: Polygonum-leaved Tabernæmontana. Hind: Tŭgŭr. A straight middling-sized tree in the gardens at Kotah: the tree is sacred, and the wood is scented and used in incense.

Tabernæmontana Coronaria: Rose-bay like Tabernæmontana. Hind: Firki-Tugur, the single-flowered, and Bŭra-Tugur, the double-flowered. Common in gardens at Kotah and elsewhere. This shrub is very ornamental and the flowers are fragrant during the night.

DIGYNIA.

Asclepias Gigantea: Great Swallow Wort. Hind: Ak; Mudar. Very common every where at Ajmeer. I have long used the powdered bark of the root as an emetic, and in indolent cutaneous diseases. In many parts of Marwar, and even at Ajmeer, the stalks of this plant are used as rafters.

Asclepias Pendula: Pendulous Swallow Wort. Cultivated in gardens at Kotah. The flowers have a pleasant odour and the plant is very hardy.

Chenopodium Viride: Green Goosefoot. Hind: Hurra-sag. The red and green variety of this is called Lál-sag. Both are cultivated by the malees as pot-herbs.

Beta Bengalensis: Bengal-Beet. Hind: Palag-sag. Cultivated in gardens for the leaves, which are used as a pot-herb, and eat very like spinach.

Beta Vulgaris: Red Beet Root. Hind: Lal Chŭkŭndŭr. } Cultivated.

Beta Cĭcla: White Beet Root. Hind: Sufaid Chŭkŭndŭr. } Cultivated.

Gomphrena Globosa: Globe Amaranth; Everlasting flower. Hind: Gool-mŭkhmul. Both red and white varieties cultivated in gardens.

Semecarpus Anacardium: Marking Nut-tree. Hind: Bhiláwan. Grows in the Kotah and Mewar jungles.

Ligusticum Ajowan: Lovage. Hind: Ajwain. Cultivated for the carminative seed.

Cuminum Cyminum: Cumin Seed. Hind: Sufaid-zeera. Cultivated for the seed.

Coriandrum Sativum: Coriander. Hind: Dhuniya, the seed; Khôt-meer, the green plant. Much cultivated as a condiment.

Anethum Sowa: Indian Fennel. Hind: Sowa. Cultivated and eaten raw with spices, or boiled as a condiment.

Apium Involucratum: Involucred Parsley. Hind: Ajmod. Cultivated for the carminative seed.

Trigynia.

Tamarix Diocca: Red Tamarisk. Hind: Lal-jhao. Very common in the beds of rivers.

Tamarix Indica: Indian Tamarisk. Hind: Ferish; Ferash; Jhao. A tree of considerable size, common in the Ajmeer district; the wood is very inferior.

Pharnaceum Mollugo: Ladies Bed Straw. Hind: Ghima-sag. Wild in gardens during the rains; sometimes used as a pot-herb.

Basella Alba: Malabar Nightshade. Hind: Poi; Bun-poi. Cultivated at Ajmeer as ornamental and as a pot-herb.

Pentagynia.

Linum Usitatissimum: Common Flax. Hind: Ulsee. Cultivated for the oil seed.

Linum Trigynum: Three-styled Flax. Hind: Gool-ashrufi. Cultivated as a flower in gardens.

Hexandria Monogynia.

Bromelia Ananas: Pine Apple. Hind: Ananas. Does not thrive at Ajmeer; and is only rarely cultivated at Kotah.

Tradescantia Imbricata: Imbricated Spider Wort. A common weed in moist places during the rains.

Crinum Asiaticum: Poison-bulb. Hind: Sookh-dursun (interview of ease). Cultivated as a lily in gardens; the flowers are fragrant; the juice of the leaves is applied to the meatus auditorius externus in ear-ache; the juice is also emetic, but is very irregular in its action.

Crinum Toxicarium. Hind: Bura-kanoor. Cultivated in gardens at Kotah and elsewhere, and is very ornamental.

Crinum Zeylanicum: Cingalese Crinum. Hind: Sookh-dursun. Grows wild in low grounds near the Chumbul river.

Amaryllis Aurea: Golden Amaryllis. Hind: Zurd-sosan. Cultivated in gardens and very ornamental.

Allium Porrum: Leek. Hind: Gundeena. Sometimes cultivated in European gardens.

Allium Cepa: Common Onion. Hind: Peeaj. Cultivated

from English seed, along with Allium Ascalonicum. The Hindoos of Rajwarra largely consume onions. Very fine onions come from Jessulmeer.

Allium Sativum: Garlic. Hind: Lusoona. Cultivated by the malees, and much consumed.

Gloriosa Superba: Superb Gloriosa. Hind: Cariari. Grows wild in the Ajmeer hills in the rains.

Scilla Montana: Hill Squill. Hind: Junglee Peeaj. Grows wild abundantly in the Ajmeer hills, and the root is used to cement the colours in dying cloth in paterns.

Asparagus Officinalis: Common Asparagus. Hind: Nakdoun. Cultivated in gardens as a vegetable

Polyanthes Tuberosa: Tube Rose. Hind: Gool-shabbo. Cultivated both single and double as a flower.

Aloe Perfoliata: Perfoliate Aloe. Hind: Guickwar; Gheekoomar. Common in and near gardens. The juice of the leaves is applied to bruises.

Hemerocallis Fulva: Narcissus of India. Hind: Nurgus; Gool-nurgus. Cultivated as a flower (Brown Day Lily). The Narcissus Fistulosus is also cultivated in European gardens.

Acorus Calamus: Sweet Flag: Indian Orris Root. Hind: Buch; Ghorbuch. Cultivated and in gardens at Kotah.

Bambusa Arundinacea: Reed Bamboo. Hind: Bans. Near the rivers in Kotah, the bamboo is abundant. This species does not grow in Ajmeer.

Bambusa Nana: Dwarf Bamboo: Hind: Puhari Bans. This is found in the Ajmeer and other Rapootanah hills; it is very strong, solid, twisted and thorny.

Digynia.

Oryza Sativa: Rice. Hind: Dhan. Wild rice grows in the Ajmeer lake, every year, on the west side. Very little is cultivated at Ajmeer. In Kotah and Mewar very fine rice is grown.

Trigynia.

Rumex Vesicarius: Bladder Sorrel. Hind: Chooka. Cultivated as a salad in some gardens.

Octandria Monogynia.

Grislea Tomentosa: Woolly Grislea. Hind: Dhawri Phool. A rare tree in Ajmeer: very ornamental both in foliage and blossom. The flowers are used in dying. This tree would do well in compounds.

This is very distinct from the Dhao, which is the common firewood of Ajmeer.

Mimusops Elengi: Pointed-leaved Mimusops. Hind: Maulsari. Thrives well at Ajmeer, growing to a large size; the flowers are delightfully fragrant, and the wood is very hard and durable, the foliage is beautiful and evergreen. The berries are eaten sometimes by the poor. This tree would be very ornamental in compounds.

Mimusops Kauki: Obtuse-leaved Mimusops. Hind: Kirine. Cultivated at Ajmeer and Kotah; the tree becomes very large and is very handsome; the small fruit is eatable; the wood is fine-grained and hard.

Amyris Commiphora. Hind: Googul; Googula. A very abundant tree and shrub in the Ajmeer hills; the tree yields a gum called googul gond, used as incense and in medicine; the gum is very like myrrh; the wood is useless except to burn, and the smoke is so pungent as to make it disagreeable to use in that way.

Amyris Acuminata: Acuminated Amyris. Amyris Nana: Dwarf Amyris.	Both abundant with several other species in the Ajmeer hills.

Ximenia Ægyptica. Hind: Hingen; Hingot. Grows in the district: the nutshell is used to make crackers of in fireworks.

Lawsonia Inermis: Henna. Hind: Mĕndi. Cultivated in gardens.

Scytalia Litchi. Hind: Litchi. Rarely cultivated in gardens at Kotah and Ajmeer: the fruit is also inferior.

Sapindus Detergens: Soap Berry. Hind: Reetah. Grows in the Kotah jungles, whence the berries are exported.

Polygonum Flaccidum: Limp Bistort. Hind: Panee-mirich. Found in the rains at the marshy side of the Poshkur lake.

Decandria Monogynia.

Bauhinia Nitida : White Bauhinia. Hind : Kana Raja. Cultivated in gardens at Kotah.

Bauhinia Variegata : Variegated Bauhinia. Hind : Kuchnar. Common at Ajmeer. When in blossom the tree is very splendid, and the fragrance delightful. The flower buds are eaten as a vegetable. This tree would be highly ornamental in compounds.

Bauhinia Racemosa : Branching Bauhinia. Hind : Ghila ; Mahwal. An extensive creeper running over trees in the Kotah jungles.

Cassia Fistula : Pipe Cassia. Hind : Amultas. Grows on a hill near Rajghur in the Ajmeer district ; a common tree or shrub in Kotah. The viscid secretion on the sepimenta of the pods is generally used as a laxative by the natives. The bark of the root is strongly purgative. This is a most elegant tree, and would be highly ornamental in compounds ; the profuse yellow blossom, is more beautiful than laburnum.

Cassia Sophera. Hind : Kasaundi. Grows wild, but is not very common : the leaves are applied pounded to the itch.

Cassia Tora. Hind : Chakūnda. Grows wild during the rains ; and is rarely met with.

Cassia Purpurea. Hind : Kala-kasaundi. Grows near houses during the rains.

Cassia Obtusifolia : Blunt-leaved Cassia. Hind : Chuḳowur ; Chukaunda ; Pōwār. Rare at Ajmeer, but very common in the black soil of Kotah. The young plants are eaten as a pot-herb.

Cassia Aurata : Golden-flowered Cassia. Hind : Turwŭr ; Aola. Very common on all the hills of Ajmeer and Mewar. This is a very ornamental bush, with large golden flowers, very handsome in the rains ; it is very abundant on the Nusseerabad road.

This plant was considered to mark the Mewar hills, and the babul the Marwar country ; hence the adage,

Bawul, Bawul, Marwar:
Aola, Aola, Mewar.

Cassia Planisiliqua: Flat-podded Cassia. Cultivated in a few gardens; is not indigenous: is of very rapid growth and the wood is hard. This tree is highly ornamental, and would much adorn compounds.

Poinciana Pulcherrima: Spanish Carnations. Hind: Crishna-churrun; Gul-i-turra. Commonly cultivated at Ajmeer; it is a splendid shrub during the rains and very hardy.

Cæsalpinia Sappan: Sappan Wood. Hind: Putunga; Săppăn. Grows in the Kotah jungles; the wood is a red dye, and is also very hard.

Cæsalpinia Bonducella: Bonduc Nut. Hind: Kutkuranja; Kutkulija. Grows in hedges near gardens at Ajmeer. The nuts and leaves are used as febrifuges by the natives.

Cæsalpinia Sepiaria: Hedge Cæsalpinia. Hind: Kilgutch. Grows in one hedge at Ajmeer. Forms a splendid impenetrable hedge, covered with bright green leaves, and large yellow spikes of flowers.

Hyperanthera Mor inga: Horse Radish-tree. Hind: Sujuna; Suhujna. Common in gardens at Ajmeer.

Gærtnera Rascmosa: Branching Gærtnera. Hind: Maltilata. A fine specimen runs over some trees in the Dowlutbagh at Ajmeer. This is a fine and fragrant flowered creeper, and very hardy.

Boswellia Thurifera: Frankincense or Olibanum-tree. Hind: Salar; Salahie. Very common on the Ajmeer hills, and elsewhere; the wood is cheap and very worthless. The tree yields abundance of gum resin; but it in not gathered or put to use at Ajmeer. The tree is very abundant, and the natives of Ajmeer call the resin "luban," from which an excellent clear turpentine might be distilled.

Buchanania Latifolia: Broad-leaved Buchanania. Hind: Piyal; Achhar; Piyala. Common in the Kotah jungles; the fruit is agreeable, and the seed is the "chironji," which is much eaten in sweetmeats, and has a very pleasant rich flavour. The tree is very handsome, the flowers fragrant, and the wood hard and durable.

Melia Azedirachta: Common Bead-tree. Hind: Neem. The most common tree in Rajwarra, next to the babool.

Melia Sempervirens: Evergreen Bead-tree. Hind: Bukain. Common at Ajmeer; as is also the large deciduous variety. This is the chief tree in compounds; being very ornamental when in blossom, and odoriferous.

Swietenia Febrifuga: Febrifuge Mahogany. Hind: Rohunna. Common in the lower parts of the hills in the Kotah jungles.

Tribulus Lanuginosus: Woolly Caltrops. Hind: Gokooroo; Gokru. Very universal over the ground in Rajwarra. The seeds and capsules are highly mucilaginous.

Feronia Elephantum: Elephant's Apple. Hind: Keitha; Kutha. Rare in Ajmeer; plentiful in Boondee and Kotah. The fruit is acid and much eaten, as a condiment, raw. The wood is very hard. The tree is very ornamental, and would be an acquisition in compounds.

Aquillaria Agallocha: Aloe Wood. Hind. Ŭggŭr. There are many large trees in the gardens at Kotah. The wood is used in incense and scents.

Terminalia Catappa: Bengal Almond. Hind: Badam. In the Kotah gardens; this is a very handsome garden tree.

Terminalia Bellerica: Belleric Myrobalan. Hind: Buhira. Abundant in the Kotah jungles; the wood is very hard.

Terminalia Chebula: Chebulic Myrobalan. Hind: Har; Harra. Common in the Kotah jungles.

Terminalia Citrina: Citron-leaved Myrobalan. Hind: Har; Harituki. Also common in the Kotah jungles.

All these Myrobalans are largely collected, and used by natives in dying and in medicine.

Digynia.

Dianthus Chinensis: Indian Pink. Common in gardens.

Dianthus Caryophyllus: Clove Gilliflower. Hind: Kurrunphool. Common, of several varieties in gardens.

Pentagynia.

Averrhoa Carambola : Cocked-hat Fruit. Hind : Kumruk. Cultivated in gardens at Jaepoor and Kotah.

Averrhoa Acida : Sour Averrhoa. Hind : Harpharewri. Wild in Kotah.

Spondias Mangifera : Hog Plum. Hind : Amra. Cultivated in gardens.

Oxalis Sensitiva : Sensitive Sorrel. Hind : Lak-chana. Common weed near hedges of gardens.

Portulaca Oleracea : Edible Purslain. Hind : Noniya. Common in gardens, wild and cultivated.

Gatæva Tapia. Garlick Pear. Hind: Burua: Very common at Ajmeer; Flowers very splendid: beads made of the Wood.

Trigynia.

Euphorbia Nereifolia : Oleander-leaved Euphorbia. Hind : Sij ; Sehund. Abundant over all the hills within some miles of Ajmeer.

Euphorbia Antiquorum : True Euphorbia. Hind : Thuar. Branches triangular. More abundant than the previous species.

An immense quantity of gum resin might be collected from both of these. The dried stalks are the cheapest firewood.

Euphorbia Thymifolia : Thyme-leaved Euphorbia. Hind : Duddhi. A very common weed every where in the plains.

Icosandria Monogynia.

Cactus Indica : Indian Cactus. Hind : Nag-phunee. Found in hedges in some gardens.

Cactus Opuntia : Prickly Pear. Hind : Bura Nag-phunee. In hedges at Kotah.

Psidium Pyriferum :
Psidium Pomiferum : } Guava. Hind : Geeaboo ; Bēheē ; Amrut ; Sufri-am. Both species culvated at Ajmeer.

Eugenia Jambolana : Eugenia. Hind : Jam ; Jamun. Cultivated in gardens, and wild in Kotah and Mewar. The wood is very durable, the fruit wholesome, and the tree very ornamental, and attains a large size.

Eugenia Jambos : Rose Apple. Hind : Golab-jamun. Cultivated in gardens.

Eugenia Caryophyllifolia : Narrow-leaved Eugenia. Hind : Chota-jam. A large tree, abundant in the Kotah jungles, near water : the wood is excellent and does not rot in water, and hence is used to line wells with.

Eugenia Paniala. Hind : Paniala Jam. A very large species not uncommon on the banks of streams in Kotah.

Myrtus Communis : Common Myrtle. Hind : Belattee Mendee. Cultivated in gardens and thrives well.

Punica Granatum : Pomegranate. Hind : Anar; Darim. This tree is common and the fruit superior in the Ajmeer gardens.

Gool-anar is the double-flowered variety, and is common.

Amygdalus Persica : Peach. Hind : Aroo. Both round and fine are cultivated ; but are not superior.

Prunus —— : Hind : Aloobokhara. } Both cultivated in
—— : Aloocha. } gardens at Ajmeer ;
they are hardy, and very beautiful from their profusion of blossom.

Alangium Decapetalum : Ten-petaled Alangium. Hind : Akol ; Akarkanta. Common in Kotah ; grows to a large size ; the blossoms in March are very fragrant ; the wood of old trees is dark and scented ; would grow easily and be ornamental in compounds.

Pentagynia.

Pyrus Communis : Pear. Hind : Nas-pattee. Cultivated in gardens.

Pyrus Malus : Apple. Hind : Seeo. Commonly cultivated and thrives well at Ajmeer.

Cydonia Tomentosa : Woolly Quince. Hind : Belattee Behee. Cultivated in some gardens.

Eriobotrya Japonica : Common Loquat. Hind : Loquat. Cultivated in gardens ; but does not thrive well.

Polygynia.

Rosa Centifolia : Hundred-leaved Rose. Hind : Desee Goolab. Very commonly cultivated.

Rosa Chinensis : China Rose. Hind : Chini Goolab. Cultivated in gardens and thrives well : also a damask variety.

Rosa Glandulifera : Gland-bearing White Rose. Hind : Sewti. Commonly cultivated in gardens, always in blossom and thrives well.

Rosa Involucrata : Involucred White Rose. Hind : Sufaid Goolab. This species flowers twice during the year, and some times every month ; and was procured by me from Lucknow. It is very like the Maiden's Blush Rose, and is beautiful and fragrant.

Rosa Bifloreus : Twice-flowering Rose : Hind : Suda Goolab ; Bhadoori Goolab. This beautiful species is the most common at Ajmeer ; the rose is large, double red, and flowers after cutting in March and April, and again without cutting in August, and in a good soil flowers constantly more or less. The sepals are exceedingly prolonged, and sometimes turn into pinnate leaves.

Rosa Alba : Single White Rose. The flower is large and pure white and was brought to Ajmeer from the hills.

Fragaria Elatior : Hautboy Strawberry. Cultivated in some gardens ; but does not thrive in this climate, which is probably too dry.

Polyandria Monogynia.

Bassia Latifolia : Broad-leaved Bassia. Hind : Mowa ; Mahúa. Common in Kotah the flowers are fermented, and a strong spirit is distilled : and oil, nearly congealed at ordinary temperatures, is expressed from the seeds ; the wood is very hard and durable ; and the tree is altogether handsome.

Diospyrus Ebenum : Ebony Tree. Hind : Tendua, the tree ; Abnous, the black heart ; Tendua, the white and spotted wood. Common in the Kotah jungles, especially near Gerdhurpoora. The young trees yield a fine-grained tough very hard wood, excellent for making hackeries, &c. &c. : the ebony is not used : the very inferior fruit is eaten, when rotted like the medlar.

Symplocos Racemosa : Racemed Symplocos. Hind : Lodh. Grows in the Kotah jungles ; the bark is used to dye red with, and is exported.

Acacia Serissa : Siris. Hind : Siris. Grows at Ajmeer ; abundant in Kotah ; a beautiful tree with very fragrant flowers ; the wood is valuable.

Acacia Scandens : Climbing Mimosa. Hind : Gila. A large creeper running over trees in the Kotah jungles, where the stems of this plant often in size and form resemble ship cables.

Acacia Arabica : Gum Arabic tree. Hind : Babul ; Kikar. Of this there are two varieties at Ajmeer ; one with erect branches, the other the common one ; these are the most common and useful trees in Rajwarra. The bark is fermented with sugar into a strong spirit, and much used in tanning.

Acacia Edula : Esculent Acacia. Hind : Khējrá. A very common large tree in Rajwarra ; the long slender pods are very sweet and pleasant food cooked ; for this purpose they are universally gathered by the poor wherever procurable, and eaten both fresh and dried. The wood is very hard ; but the tree is not cut down.

Acacia (Rewa) : Sacred Acacia. Hind : Rewa. A large tree common in Rajwarra, sacred to the Matajee, around whose shrines groves of this tree are commonly found. The wood is hard, dark-coloured, and durable, but only the decayed trees are used.

Acacia (Rheonj) : Traveller's Acacia. Hind : Rheonj. A very common tree in particular parts of Rajwarra, upon which travellers at certain parts of the roads suspend shreds of their clothes (as in other parts of India). To the extremities of the young branches are suspended innumerable masses of exuded sap of large size.

Acacia (Choŭkŭr) : A species of Silk Tree Acacia. Hind: Choŭkŭr. A common low tree in many parts of Rajwarra. The flowers are long, cylindrical, one-half yellow, the other half bright pink, and not mutable, the coloured stamina exactly resembles tufts of floss silk, the wood is put to no use.

Acacia Faruesiana: Scented Babool: West Indian Sponge tree. Hind: Gooya Babula: Dukhuni Babool. Common at Ajmeer in garden hedges; grows to the size of a large bush.

Acacia Catechu: Catechu tree. Hind: Keir; Khair; Khaira. Common in the Ajmeer jungles. Kuth or Catechu is not extracted.

Acacia Suma. Hind: Sai-kanta. Common wherever there is hill jungle in Ajmeer.

Acacia Pinnata: Winged Acacia. Hind: Biswool. Rare in the Ajmeer jungles.

Mimosa Pudica: Sensitive plant. Hind: Lajuk. Cultivated in gardens.

Mimosa Concinna: Neat Mimosa. Hind: Chota Lajuk. Cultivated in flower pots.

Capparis Kurēla: Common Wild Caper tree. Hind: Kurēla. Very common everywhere in Rajwarra; and often becomes a considerable tree in the jungles: the flowers are red and very handsome; one species has yellow flowers.

Papaver Somniferum: Poppy. Hind: Post. Largely cultivated of various colours: much opium made.

Argemone Mexicana: Thorny Poppy. Hind: Sheal-kanta. Very common everywhere. The seeds are neither narcotic, nor emetic at Ajmeer.

Nymphæa Rosacea: Pink Water-lily. Hind: Rŭktă Kŭmbŭlă. Cultivated in tanks, and also wild at Poshkur, &c.

Nymphæa Lotus: White Water-lily. Hind: Koee; Kumooda; Kumul. At Poshkur, Sambhur, &c.

Nymphæa Cyanea: Blue Lotus. Hind: Neel-Pudma. In the Poshkur lake.

Œgle Marmelos: Bengal Quince. Hind. Bēlă; Bĭlvă. Common in the jungles, especially at Kotah. The large fruited sort is cultivated. This tree would be ornamental and thrive well in compounds.

Bixa Orellana: Annotta tree. Hind: Lutkun. Is found in the Kotah jungles; but, I do not believe that the pods are gathered for use.

Grewia Asiatica. Hind: Phulsa. Cultivated at Ajmeer; both large tree and small bush varieties. The large tree is very beautiful when in new foliage.

Mesua Ferrea. Hind: Nag-kesur. Cultivated in gardens at Jaepoor; is very ornamental, and the flowers are fragrant.

Shorea Robusta. Hind: Sal; Sankho. Abundant in the Kotah jungles.

Garcinia Cowa. Hind: Kowa. Common near water in Kotah and Mewar and attains a very large size: yields a gum resin like gamboge; which however is not collected.

Pentagynia.

Nigella Indica: Indian Fennel Flower. Hind: Kala-zira. Cultivated and wild in the district.

Dillenia Speciosa. Hind: Gĭrnār. This beautiful tree is abundant in the Kotah jungles: the very large bright yellow blossoms are most magnificent. This tree would be exceedingly ornamental in compounds, and would thrive well, being very hardy.

Michelia Chumpaca: Chumpa. Hind: Chumpa. Cultivated for its fragrant flowers: it is a beautiful tree; the fruit is not eaten.

Annona Squamosa: Custard apple. Hind: Sita-phul; Shureefa; Ata. Cultivated at Ajmeer; but the fruit is inferior.

Didynamia Gymnospermia.

Mentha Sativa: Garden Mint. Hind: Podeena. Cultivated and thrives well.

Mentha Viridis: Spear Mint. Hind: Belatti Podeena. Cultivated in gardens.

Ocymum Villosum: Woolly Basil. Hind: Sufaid Toolsi. Cultivated in gardens and near temples.

Ocymum Sanctum: Holy Basil. Hind: Kala Toolsi. Cultivated near temples.

Ocymum Pilosum: Hairy Basil. Hind: Babai; Babooi Toolsi. Very common as a weed over all Rajwarra. The green leaves have a delicious smell, exactly like verbena: the seeds are exceedingly mucilaginous, and sometimes used as a demulcent. The dried plant prevents bugs approaching beds, &c.

Ocymum Gratissimum: Strong-scented Basil. Hind: Ram Toolsi. Cultivated near temples.

Plectranthus Aromaticus: Fragrant Plectranthus. Hind: Pathur-choor. Cultivated in gardens at Ajmeer.

Vitex Trifolia: Three-leaved Chaste tree. Hind: Samalū. Grows wild and is also cultivated in some places.

Vitex Negundo: Blue-flowered Chaste tree. Hind: Nisinda. Cultivated in gardens at Ajmeer as ornamental.

Celsia Asiatica: Indian Celsia. Hind: Kookshima. A common weed in gardens.

Ses-amum Orientale: Indian Ses-amum. Hind: Til. Both white and dark seeded varieties are cultivated; but do not thrive well.

Bignonia Undulata: Waved-leaved Bignonia. Hind: Rohira; Reôra. A very common tree in Marwar and other parts of Rajwarra. This tree when covered, in the month of March, with its immense quantities of orange-coloured blossoms is a most splendid object, and would be highly ornamental in compounds: the wood is fine-grained and valuable, having a scent like the walnut leaf.

Bignonia Surberosa: Cork-barked Bignonia. Hind: Neemi Chambeli. In gardens at Ajmeer. This beautiful tree is a very rapid grower. The rough bark peels off in small pieces about once a year. In January the tree is covered with blossoms, which are beautiful and fragrant in a high degree.

Tetradynamia Siliculosa.

Lepidium Sativum: Common Cresses. Hind: Halim. Cultivated in gardens.

Brassica Rapa: Turnip. Hind: Shulgam.

Brassica Oleracea: Cabbage. Hind: Gobee; Cauliflower, Phool-gobee; Knole-kole, Gânth-gobee. All varieties cultivated and thrive well.

N. B. In Rajwarra the Hindoos, both rich and poor, eat turnips, carrots and cabbages, besides onions; having no prejudices in this respect regarding caste.

Sinapis Dichotomus: Two-branched Mustard. Hind: Soorsun Rai. Cultivated for the seed.

Sinapis Glauca: Hoary Mustard. Hind: Sufaid Rai. Also cultivated.

Raphanus Sativus: Radish. Hind: Moolee. Much cultivated and attain a large size.

Cleome Viscosa: Viscid Cleome. Hind: Hoorhooriya. This is a very common annual weed in Rajwarra, especially at Ajmeer: the plant has a very strong nauseous smell: the seeds are eaten in curries.

MONADELPHIA PENTANDRIA.

Pistia Stratioites. Hind: Takie-panie. A weed found floating in the Ajmeer lake, after a heavy rainy season.

DODECANDRIA.

Helicteres Isora: Screw plant. Hind: Marôr-phulli. All names of the same meaning. Cultivated in gardens. Is like the phulsa in foliage. The natives have an absurd idea that this plant benefits in cholics, owing to some sympathy with the twisted nature of the pods.

Sterculia Urens: Stinging Sterculia. Hind: Kur; Kutila. Common in the Ajmeer hills; and in Kotah. It grows to a very large size, forming an immense tree. The kutila gond, exactly similar to gum tragacanth, is obtained in great abundance from this tree: the seeds of the stinging pods are palatable when roasted and very wholesome: many bushels must be yielded by one large tree, and the poor in famines should collect the seeds for food: the star-shaped pods are covered with stinging pubescence.

Sterculia Parviflora: Small-flowered Sterculia. Abundant in the jungles.

Bombax Heptaphylla: Seven-leaved Bombax. Hind: Sémăl. Common and of large size in the Kotah jungles and elsewhere.

Althæa Rosea: Holly-hock. Hind: Gool-khairū. Common in gardens, and inferior.

Malva Communis: Common Mallow. Hind: Chota Goolkhairū. Common in gardens, and difficult to eradicate.

Gossypium Arboreum: Tree Cotton. Hind: Bura-kupas. Cultivated in some gardens; the large yellow flowers being very ornamental.

Gossypium Herbaceum: Herbaceous Cotton. Hind: Kupas; Rui; Bun. Very inferior varieties are grown in Ajmeer: a better sort comes from Mewar and Kotah.

Gossypium Religiosum: Holy Cotton. Hind: Jŭnŭa-kupas. This red-flowered variety is cultivated in gardens: the Jŭnŭa threads worn by brahmuns, rajpoots and some of the byess tribes, are made of this Cotton.

Hibiscus Rosa Sinensis: Shoe-flower. Hind: Juva. Common in gardens. There are several varieties. The flowers at Madras are often used to clean shoes with.

Hibiscus Mutabilis: Changeable Hibiscus. Hind: Gajuba. Cultivated in gardens; the large double variety.

Hibiscus Abelmoschus: Musk Okro. Hind: Kala-kustoora. Grows wild in the rains.

Hibiscus Syriacus: Syrian Hibiscus. Hind: Gajuba. The large double pink-flowered variety is cultivated, and very common in gardens at Ajmeer.

Hibiscus Subdariffa: Hemp Hibiscus. Hind: Pŭtŭa; Putsun. Cultivated in gardens for the calices used in tarts and preserves.

Hibiscus Cannabinus: Hemp Hibiscus. Hind: Pāt-sūn. Cultivated for the fibres.

Hibiscus Esculentus: Okru; Okro. Hind: Bhindi; Ram Turai. Much cultivated as a vegetable.

DIADELPHIA TRIANDRIA.

Tamarindus Indica: Tamarind tree. Hind; Imli. Very common and of large size at Ajmeer.

HEXANDRIA.

Fumaria Parviflora: Small-flowered Fumitory. Hind: Bun-Sulpa. Common, cultivated in gardens at Ajmeer.

DECANDRIA.

Dalbergia Sissoo: Sissoo tree. Hind: Sissoo; Seesum. Scarce in the hills of Ajmeer: more abundant in Kotah. The wood of the Ajmeer tree is very dark and beautifully veined, like rose wood.

Butea Frondosa: Branching Butea. Hind: Dâk; Palas. Common in some parts of Ajmeer, and very common in Boondee and Kotah. Indian Kino, called chuni-gond, is collected from this tree. The dried flowers are called tēsū, and are used in dying.

Abrus Precatorius; Wild Liquorice. Hind: Ghoonchi. Common in the Ajmeer hills. The root dug up in the rains is very like liquorice, and very succulent: at other seasons it is hard and tasteless. Both red and white seeded varieties are common.

Crotalaria Juncea: Rush-like Hemp. Hind: Phool-sun. Cultivated for the hemp it yields. The young flowers are eaten by the poor; they are also beautiful and fragrant.

Arachis Hypogea: Indian Earth Nut. Hind: Moong-phulli. This common, but curious plant is cultivated in some places for the seeds, which are roasted and eaten as a delicacy, and are generally sold in the Ajmeer bazars.

Carpopogon Pruriens: Cowhage. Hind: Kiwanch. Common in the hills and hedges.

Phaseolus Nanus: Dwarf Kidney Bean. Hind: Frāsh-bean. Cultivated.

Phaseolus Mūngŏ: Green Gram. Hind: Moong ka dal. Cultivated in the rains wherever the soil will permit.

Phaseolus Max: Black Gram. Hind: Oord ka dal; Kalamoong. Cultivated in the same way.

Phaseolus Aconitifolius: Aconite-leaved Bean. Hind: Môth ka dal. Very generally cultivated in poor soil throughout Rajwarra: in favourable seasons the produce is great, the plant then spreading extensively. The seed is the common dâl of the poor in Rajwarra, and is also much used for horses both plain, ground, and boiled, during the cold season. It has rather a bitter taste.

Dolichos Gladiatus: Sword-podded Dolichos. Hind: Mukhun-shim. Both red and white flowered are cultivated.

Dolichos Virosus: Poisonous Dolichos. Hind: Kala-shim. Wild in hedges; but is not eaten: is very bitter; but probably not poisonous.

Dolichos Sinensis: Chinese Dolichos. Hind: Lobiya. Much cultivated as a vegetable legumen.

Dolichos Tetragonolobus: Square-lobed Dolichos. Hind. Choukona-shim. Cultivated and is an excellent vegetable.

Dolichos Phaseoloides. Kidney Bean: Dolichos. Hind: Bur-shim. Perennial. Cultivated in gardens; the pods sliced are a very good vegetable.

Clitorea Ternatea: Ternate Clitorea. Hind: Uparagita; Kowa; Kowa-theti (Crow's-beak). A common wild creeper during the rains.

Pisum Sativum: Pea. Hind: Mutur. Cultivated of various kinds in gardens and fields.

Lathyrus Alphaca: Yellow Vetchling. Hind: Massoor-chŭna. Cultivated for the grain.

Cicer Arietinum: Chick Pea. Hind: Chenna; Dana. Little cultivated in Ajmeer; but plentiful in Kotah, Boondee and Mewar.

Cicer Lens. Hind: Mussoor ka dal. Cultivated for the red grain it yields, which is preferred as a dâl by many.

Cytisus Cajan: Pigeon Pea. Hind: Urhur ka dal. The climate of Ajmeer is too cold for this grain, the frosts killing the plant; but in Kotah it is much cultivated.

whole plant is used in fevers, as elsewhere in India; every part is very bitter; an extract is prepared, called Giloysut, from the stems and leaves.

Menispermum Verrucosum: Warty-stemmed Moon-seed. Found in the Ajmeer hills.

Menispermum Cordifolium: Heart-leaved Moon-seed. Very common in the Ajmeer hills; both these plants are also called Gulancha by the natives indifferently.

Menispermum Villosum: Woolly Moon-seed. Found in the Ajmeer hills.

I only obtained one specimen of a plant, which I am almost sure was the Coculus Indicus or Plunkenetii; but I could not again obtain portions of the plant; the person who first brought it, having forgotten where he first found it.

Decandria.

Carica Papaya: Papaw tree. Hind: Papya. Cultivated at Ajmeer.

Rottlera Tinctoria. Hind: Poonag. In the Kotah jungles, and in Mewar.

Flacourtia Cataphracta: Many-spined Flacourtia. Hind: Paniyala. A fruit tree in gardens at Kotah.

FINIS.

Æschynomene Grandiflora: Great-flowered Æschynomene. Hind: Agust; Agusti; Gool-phunoos. Cultivated in gardens.

Æschynomene Sesban. Hind: Jait; Jyunti. Common in hedges and gardens.

Hedysarum Alhagi: Prickly-stemmed Hedysarum. Hind: Jŭwāsă. Very common every where in Rajwarra.

Hedysarum Junceum: Rush-stemmed Hedysarum. Grows in vast quantities in Shekhawattie and elsewhere, near Jaepore: the small branches are sweet and eaten by camels and other cattle. This becomes a considerable bush, and has no thorns.

Indigofera Cærulea: Puce-flowered Indigo. Hind: Lil. Very common all over the Ajmeer district, often covering the whole country.

Indigofera Fragrans: Scented Indigo. Is rare in the Ajmeer district.

Indigofera Tinctoria: Dye Indigo. Cultivated, and also wild.

Trigonella Fœnumgræcum: Fenugreek. Hind: Methee. Cultivated as a pot-herb, and for the seed.

Trifolium Indicum: Indian Trefoil. Hind: Bun-methee; Jhoonjoorie; Goolalie. Very common in Ajmeer, Marwar and Jaepoor. Camels are fond of it; other cattle do not eat it.

Polyadelphia Icosandria.

Citus Acida: Lime; Lemon. Hind: Neeboo. Both limes and lemons are cultivated at Ajmeer.

Citrus Aurantium: Orange. Hind: Narangie; Cintra. The Ajmeer oranges are scarce and bad. Those of Kotah and Tonk are excellent and abundant.

Citrus Medica: Citron. Hind: Kurua-neeboo; Bejoura. Cultivated; the long sort scarce; the round sort abundant.

Citrus Decumana: Shaddock. Hind: Chakotara; Batabee-neeboo. Rarely cultivated.

Syngenesia Æqualis.

Lactuca Sativa. Lettuce. Hind : Khos ; Salad. Cultivated in gardens.

Serratula Anthelmintica : Worm Saw-wort. Hind : Somraj. Grows wild in Kotah.

Carthamus Tinctorius : Officinal Carthamus ; Safflower. Hind : Koosum. Cultivated on a small scale.

Superflua.

Artemisia Indica : Indian Wormwood. Hind : Dona ; Gundmar. Common in native gardens.

Artemisia Sternutatoria : Errhine Wormwood : Hind : Nakchiknee. A small plant found in the fields that have been cultivated.

Aster Chinensis : Chinese Star Flower. Very common in gardens.

Tagetes Patula : French Mary-gold. Hind : Gool-jafari. Common in gardens.

Tagetes Erecta : Tall Mary-gold. Hind : Genda. A great variety in gardens.

Chrysanthemum Indicum : Indian Chrysanthemum. Hind : Gool-daoodi. Yellow and white varities are common.

Eclipta Prostrata : Trailing Eclipta. Hind : Bhangi Keysuti. A common weed in the rains.

Helianthus Annuus : Sun-flower. Hind : Suraj-mukhi. Very common in gardens.

Helianthus Tuberosus : Jerusalem Artichoke. Cultivated in gardens.

Centaurea Moschata : Musk Centaury. Hind : Sha-pusund. Cultivated as a flower.

Sphæranthus Mollis : Soft Globe-flower. Hind : Gork-mundi. Common near the Ana-sagur ; used by the natives in medicine.

Echinops Echinatus : Camel Thistle. Hind : Oont-katara. Very common in Rajwarra ; camels consume it readily.

Monœcia Monandria.

Arum Colocasia : Edible Arum. Hind : Kuchoo; Ghoya. Commonly cultivated for the tuberous roots, which are however very indigestible.

Arum Indicum : Indian Arum. Hind : Bura-kuchoo ; Mankuchoo. Cultivated at Kotah ; the stalks and roots are eaten.

Arum Campanulatum : Campanulate Arum. Hind : Jemkund ; Ol. Found wild in the jungles. The root is very large and is eaten boiled or roasted. It is very acrid when raw.

Artocarpus Integrifolia : Jack Fruit-tree ; Entire-leaved Bread Fruit-tree. Hind : Kutul ; Kuthol. Cultivated in Kotah gardens.

Artocarpus Lakoocha. Hind : Burhul. Also cultivated at Kotah for the fruit.

Ficus Carica : Fig. Hind : Unjeer. At Ajmeer there are three varieties of figs cultivated ; one, the Turkey fig, was introduced by me.

Ficus Indica : Banyan-tree. Hind : Bur ; Burgud. Wild, of large size, near tanks and villages.

Ficus Religiosa : Sacred Fig-tree. Hind : Peepul. Found in the same situations as the above.

Ficus Infectoria : Vein-leaved Fig-tree. Hind : Pakur. More rarely met with than the two former.

Ficus Glomerata : Bunched Fig-tree. Hind : Goolar ; Doombar. Common near water.

Triandria.

Zea Mays : Indian Corn. Hind : Mŭkkă ; Bhŭtă. Much cultivated as a grain, in Ajmeer : eaten both green and ground into flour.

Tetrandria.

Morus Alba :
Morus Atropurpurea : } Mulberry. Hind : Sha-toot. Cultivated in gardens ; the fruit is very inferior.

PENTANDRIA.

Amaranthus Polygamus : Hermaphrodite Amaranth. Hind : Chaulai. Very common as a weed at Ajmeer. The leaves are eaten by the poor as a pot-herb. It is also cultivated. Where the soil is very poor, this plant becomes thorny.

Amaranthus Viridis : Green Amaranth. Hind : Hurra-sag. Cultivated as a pot-herb.

Amaranthus Lividus : Red Amaranth. Hind : Lal-sag. Much cultivated as a pot-herb.

Amaranthus Gangeticus : Bengal Amaranth. Hind : Lal-sag. Less red than the preceding ; also cultivated.

HEXANDRIA.

Areca Gracilis : Slender Areca. Hind : Gooa-supiyari. A rare tree in the gardens at Kotah.

POLYANDRIA.

Aleurites Triloba : Bengal Walnut. Hind : Akroot. A fruit tree in the Kotah gardens ; the fruit is similar in flavour to the walnut.

MONADELPHIA.

Cupressus Sempervirens : Cypress. Hind : Săräss. In gardens at Ajmeer and Kotah.

Phyllanthus Emblica : Emblic Myrobalan. Hind : Aola ; Anola. In gardens at Ajmeer, and wild in Kotah and Mewar.

Phyllanthus Longifolius : Cheramella. Hind : Harpharewri. In gardens and wild in Kotah : the acid berry is eaten.

Croton Tiglium : Croton. Hind : Jemalgota, the seed, and also Jayapala ; the root is called Duntărī. Grows wild in Kotah and Mewar ; the seeds are small and little used.

Jatropha Curcas : Angular-leaved Physic-nut. Hind : Bhagbarinda ; Bhagarendi. Common in garden hedges in Kotah.

Ricinus Communis: Castor Oil-tree. Hind: Arendi; Irrun; Rendi. Commonly cultivated everywhere near houses.

SYNGENESIA.

Trichosanthes Diœca: Diœcious Snake Gourd. Hind: Pulwul. Both wild and cultivated in the rains.

Trichosanthes Anguina: Snake Gourd. Hind: Chichinga; Chichinda. Cultivated in the rains.

Momordica Charanthia: Hairy Momordica. Hind: Kurēla. Cultivated in the rains.

Momordica Muricata. Hind: Bura Kurēla. Also cultivated.

Luffa Pentandra: Five-stamined Luffa. Hind: Gheeaturai. Much cultivated in the rains.

Luffa Acutangula: Angular-fruited Luffa. Hind: Chaulaturai. Much cultivated in the rains.

Cucurbita Lagenaria: Bottle Gourd. Hind: Tomra; Kudoo. Different varieties are cultivated.

Cucurbita Pepo. Pumpkin. Hind: Koomroo; Kudima. Large and small varieties much cultivated; the kudima is a sweet kind. Petha is the long white variety.

Cucurbita Melopepo: Squash. Hind: Khakhor. Cultivated over the malees' houses in the rains. In Bengal this is called Suphura-koomra.

Cucurbita Citrullus: Water Melon. Hind: Turbooza. Very fine cultivated ones in Ajmeer; and wild in Marwar and Beekaneer.

Cucumis Colocynthis: Colocynth. Hind: Indrayan. Common, wild, in fruit in November, all over Ajmeer and Jaepoor; Buffaloes eat the bitter fruit with apparent zest, and uninjured.

Cucumis Melo: Melon. Hind: Kurbooza. Commonly cultivated; but, not superior in Ajmeer. Two delicious small varieties of melon grow wild in Marwar, Beekaneer and Jessulmeer; they are very small and high-flavoured, and are exported as delicacies. Probably the Cucumis Madraspatanus (Hind: Bun-gunuk) and the Cucumis Turbinatus (Hind: Kachari.)

Cucumis Sativus: Cucumber. Hind: Keera. Cultivated in the rains.

Cucumis Momordica. Hind: Phoont; Tooti. Cultivated and wild in the rains.

Cucumis Utilissimus. Hind: Kakri. Abundantly cultivated in the hot winds.

Diœcia Monandria.

Pandanus Odoratissimus: Green-spined Screw Pine. Hind: Kateki; Ketki; Keora. The white-flowered variety is called Keora, and the yellow-flowered variety, Ketki. Both are abundant near Ajmeer, and of large size near water in the valleys, and also in Kotah.

Diandria.

Salix Babylonica: Weeping Willow. Hind: Bêt mujuee; Leilie-Mujnoo. Cultivated in gardens at Ajmeer.

Pentandria.

Spinacia Tetrandra: Spinach. Hind: Pinach. Cultivated as a pot-herb.

Cannabis Sativa: Hemp. Hind: Bhang; Ganja. Very common in Ajmeer, both wild and cultivated as an intoxicating drug.

Hexandria.

Phœnix Sylvestris: Date-tree. Hind: Khujoor. Grows wild in some parts of Rajwarra.

Phœnix Dactylifera: Eatable Date-tree. In a garden at Ajmeer; and said to grow near Jessulmeer.

Borassus Flabelliformis: Fan Palm. Hind: Tar; Tal. A rare tree in Rajwarra; but is seen in Ajmeer and in Boondee.

Dioscorea Alata: Winged Plantain. Hind: Rat-alū. Cultivated; but the roots are inferior.

Dioscorea Purpurea. Cultivated in the same way.

Menispermum Glabrum: Smooth Moon-seed. Hind: Nimgĭlō. So named from its frequently growing upon Neem-trees. Hind: Gulancha. Common in Ajmeer. The

Cucumis Sativus: Cucumber. Hind: Keera. Cultivated in the rains.

Cucumis Momordica. Hind: Phoont; Tooti. Cultivated and wild in the rains.

Cucumis Utilissimus. Hind: Kakri. Abundantly cultivated in the hot winds.

Diœcia Monandria.

Pandanus Odoratissimus: Green-spined Screw Pine. Hind: Kateki; Ketki; Keora. The white-flowered variety is called Keora, and the yellow-flowered variety, Ketki. Both are abundant near Ajmeer, and of large size near water in the valleys, and also in Kotah.

Diandria.

Salix Babylonica: Weeping Willow. Hind: Bêt mujuee; Leilie-Mujnoo. Cultivated in gardens at Ajmeer.

Pentandria.

Spinacia Tetrandra: Spinach. Hind: Pinach. Cultivated as a pot-herb.

Cannabis Sativa: Hemp. Hind: Bhang; Ganja. Very common in Ajmeer, both wild and cultivated as an intoxicating drug.

Hexandria.

Phœnix Sylvestris: Date-tree. Hind: Khujoor. Grows wild in some parts of Rajwarra.

Phœnix Dactylifera: Eatable Date-tree. In a garden at Ajmeer; and said to grow near Jessulmeer.

Borassus Flabelliformis: Fan Palm. Hind: Tar; Tal. A rare tree in Rajwarra; but is seen in Ajmeer and in Boondee.

Dioscorea Alata: Winged Plantain. Hind: Rat-alū. Cultivated; but the roots are inferior.

Dioscorea Purpurea. Cultivated in the same way.

Menispermum Glabrum: Smooth Moon-seed. Hind: Nimgĭlō. So named from its frequently growing upon Neem-trees. Hind: Gulancha. Common in Ajmeer. The

Ricinus Communis: Castor Oil-tree. Hind: Arendi; Irrun; Rendi. Commonly cultivated everywhere near houses.

SYNGENESIA.

Trichosanthes Diœca: Diœcious Snake Gourd. Hind: Pulwul. Both wild and cultivated in the rains.

Trichosanthes Anguina: Snake Gourd. Hind: Chichinga; Chichinda. Cultivated in the rains.

Momordica Charanthia: Hairy Momordica. Hind: Kurēla. Cultivated in the rains.

Momordica Muricata. Hind: Bura Kurēla. Also cultivated.

Luffa Pentandra: Five-stamined Luffa. Hind: Gheeaturai. Much cultivated in the rains.

Luffa Acutangula: Angular-fruited Luffa. Hind: Chaulaturai. Much cultivated in the rains.

Cucurbita Lagenaria: Bottle Gourd. Hind: Tomra; Kudoo. Different varieties are cultivated.

Cucurbita Pepo. Pumpkin. Hind: Koomroo; Kudima. Large and small varieties much cultivated; the kudima is a sweet kind. Petha is the long white variety.

Cucurbita Melopepo: Squash. Hind: Khakhor. Cultivated over the malees' houses in the rains. In Bengal this is called Suphura-koomra.

Cucurbita Citrullus: Water Melon. Hind: Turbooza. Very fine cultivated ones in Ajmeer; and wild in Marwar and Beekaneer.

Cucumis Colocynthis: Colocynth. Hind: Indrayan. Common, wild, in fruit in November, all over Ajmeer and Jaepoor; Buffaloes eat the bitter fruit with apparent zest, and uninjured.

Cucumis Melo: Melon. Hind: Kurbooza. Commonly cultivated; but, not superior in Ajmeer. Two delicious small varieties of melon grow wild in Marwar, Beekaneer and Jessulmeer; they are very small and high-flavoured, and are exported as delicacies. Probably the Cucumis Madraspatanus (Hind: Bun-gunuk) and the Cucumis Turbinatus (Hind: Kachari.)